Inhalation therapy for pulmonary hypertension

Inhalation therapy for pulmonary hypertension

The Proceedings of a Symposium held at the
Annual Congress of the European Respiratory Society

Berlin, September 2001

Edited by

Timothy Higenbottam and Celia Emery

University of Sheffield Medical School, Sheffield, UK

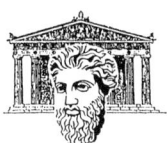

The Parthenon Publishing Group
International Publishers in Medicine, Science & Technology

A CRC PRESS COMPANY

BOCA RATON   LONDON   NEW YORK   WASHINGTON, D.C.

Schering AG have provided an educational grant to support the publication of this book.

The European Respiratory Society declines all responsibility with respect to the information published in this document.

Published in the USA by
The Parthenon Publishing Group
345 Park Avenue South, 10th Floor
New York, NY 10010
USA

Published in the UK and Europe by
The Parthenon Publishing Group
23–25 Blades Court
Deodar Road
London SW15 2NU
UK

Library of Congress Cataloging-in-Publication Data
Data available on request

British Library Cataloguing in Publication Data
Inhalation therapy for pulmonary hypertension : the
    proceedings of a symposium held at the Annual Congress of
    the European Respiratory Society, Berlin, September 2001
    1. Pulmonary hypertension - Treatment - Congresses
    2. Respiratory therapy - Congresses
    I. Higenbottam, T. II. Emery, Celia III. European Respiratory
    Society. Congress (2001 : Berlin, Germany)
    616.2'4

ISBN 1-84214-184-8

First published in 2003

Composition by The Parthenon Publishing Group
Printed and bound by Bookcraft (Bath) Ltd., Midsomer Norton, UK

Contents

List of principal contributors

Celia Emery
Division of Clinical Sciences (South)
Floor F
University of Sheffield Medical School
Beech Hill Road
Sheffield S10 2DU
United Kingdom

Nazzareno Galiè
Institute of Cardiology
University of Bologna
Via Massarenti 9
I-40138 Bologna
Italy

Timothy Higenbottam
Division of Clinical Sciences (South)
Floor F
University of Sheffield Medical School
Beech Hill Road
Sheffield S10 2DU
United Kingdom

Robert Naeije
Laboratoire de Physiologie et
   Physiopathologie
Faculty of Medicine
ULB-Hopital Erasme
Route de Lennik 808-CP604
B-1070 Brussels
Belgium

Horst Olschewski
Internal Medicine
Medical Clinic II
Universitätsklinikum Giessen
Klinikstrasse 36
D-35385 Giessen
Germany

Werner Seeger
Internal Medicine
Medical Clinic II
Universitätsklinikum Giessen
Klinikstrasse 36
D-35385 Giessen
Germany

Gerald Simonneau
Department of Pulmonary Vascular
   Diseases
Antoine Béclère Hospital
University of South Paris
Clamart
France

Preface

During the past 20 years, there has been an enormous change in the care of patients with primary pulmonary hypertension. A decade ago, it would have been very difficult to foresee that so many different treatments for this condition would have become available. This volume provides a summary of a Symposium that was a landmark meeting, presenting for the first time the results of the Aerosolized Iloprost Randomized Study in Primary and Non-Primary Pulmonary Hypertension (the AIR study). The term non-primary pulmonary hypertension (nPPH) is introduced in this volume to distinguish primary pulmonary hypertension (PPH) from other forms.

In 1998, the World Health Organization organized a consensus meeting at which a new classification of pulmonary hypertension was presented. This identified types of pulmonary hypertension in which prostanoid therapy is effective – pulmonary arterial hypertension in all its forms, and pulmonary hypertension with chronic thromboembolic disease. Now, with inhaled prostanoids, patients with hypoxic pulmonary hypertension may also be helped.

We must recall the landmarks in advances in the understanding and treatment of the disorder. These will be presented in the following chapters, which deal with the pathophysiology of the disease and its treatments, discussing the use of both prostanoid and alternative therapies and highlighting the benefit of inhaled therapy.

The reader is provided with a complete review of the state of art in the care of primary pulmonary hypertension and all other forms of pulmonary hypertension.

Timothy Higenbottam
Celia Emery

1

Prostanoid therapy for pulmonary hypertension

Timothy Higenbottam

It was 18 years ago that the present author and Lewis J. Rubin first used intravenous prostanoid therapy for primary pulmonary hypertension (PPH)[1,2]. With the realization that medical therapy was effective in this usually fatal disease, a range of novel medical therapies has now been tested.

The main focus of this meeting was to look at ways in which we can simplify the treatment of patients with PPH.

WHY PROSTANOIDS?

It is important, first, to review the reasons why the prostanoids, namely, prostacyclin and iloprost, are considered to be so important in this disease. The aims of management are principally to improve survival, as this illness, if untreated, is life-threatening. The 5-year survival of patients with untreated disease is less than 20%[3] (Figure 1).

The pathology, which is described in detail in Chapter 2, was known to involve progressive narrowing of small peripheral arteries within the acini. This contributed to a massive increase in resistance to the flow of blood through the lung. The pathophysiology of the condition involves endothelial dysfunction, leading to increased production of endothelin-1 and reduced production of the vasodilators and antiplatelet aggregating agents nitric oxide and prostacyclin (Figure 2). Indeed, detailed immunohistochemistry studies of patients with PPH (Figure 3) have shown that, in the muscular and important small arteries, there is under-expression of the enzyme that produces prostacyclin[4]. In addition to these changes, there are further pathological changes (Figure 4) suggesting intravascular thrombosis, with eccentric narrowing, both of which are features commonly found in PPH patients, compared with controls, but are also found in other forms of pulmonary hypertension, including the Eisenmenger syndrome[5].

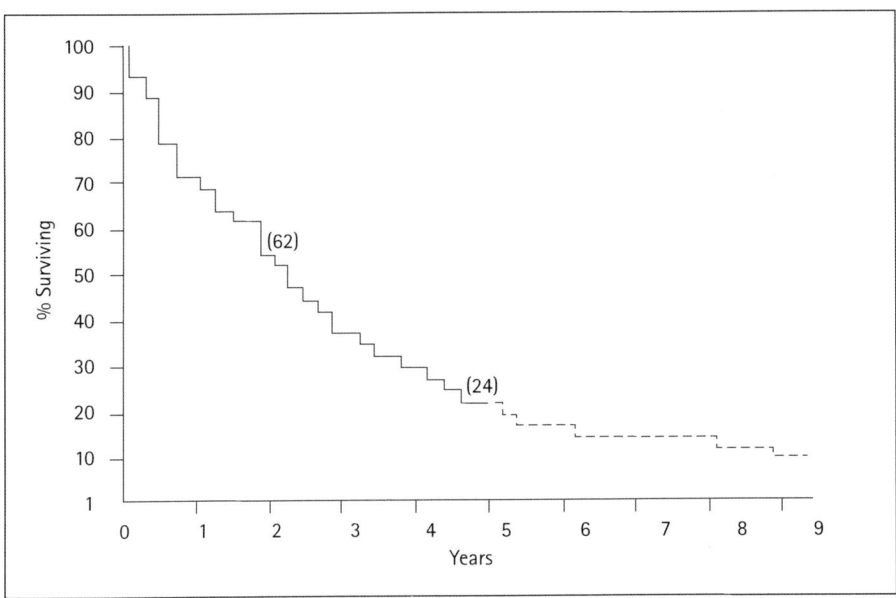

FIGURE 1   Survival curve for untreated primary pulmonary hypertension[1]

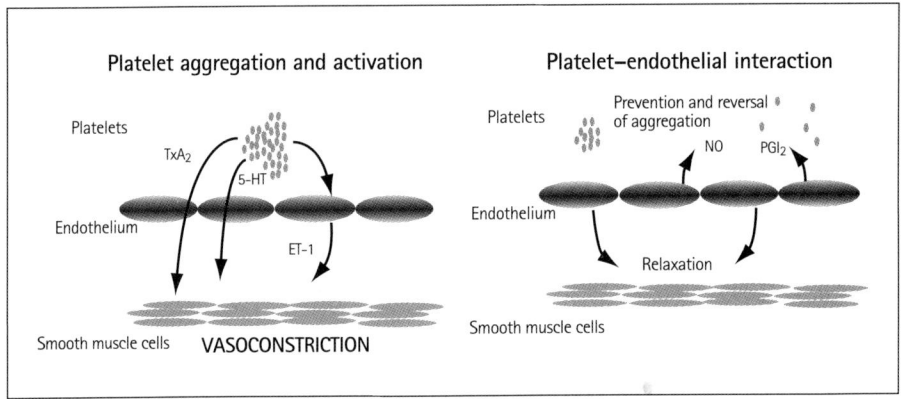

FIGURE 2   Schematic showing the changes that occur in the blood vessels with pulmonary hypertension

These changes lead to a disease which causes death as a result of right ventricular failure. Indeed, the signs which indicate a poor prognosis in such patients are a low cardiac index and elevated right atrial pressure[6] (Tables 1 and 2). These are the hallmarks of advancing disease. The reason that prostacyclin looked so attractive 18 years ago was that it is a powerful vasodilator, leading to increased cardiac output, and it is not associated with elevation of right atrial pressure (unpublished). In addition, it has the added benefit of inhibiting

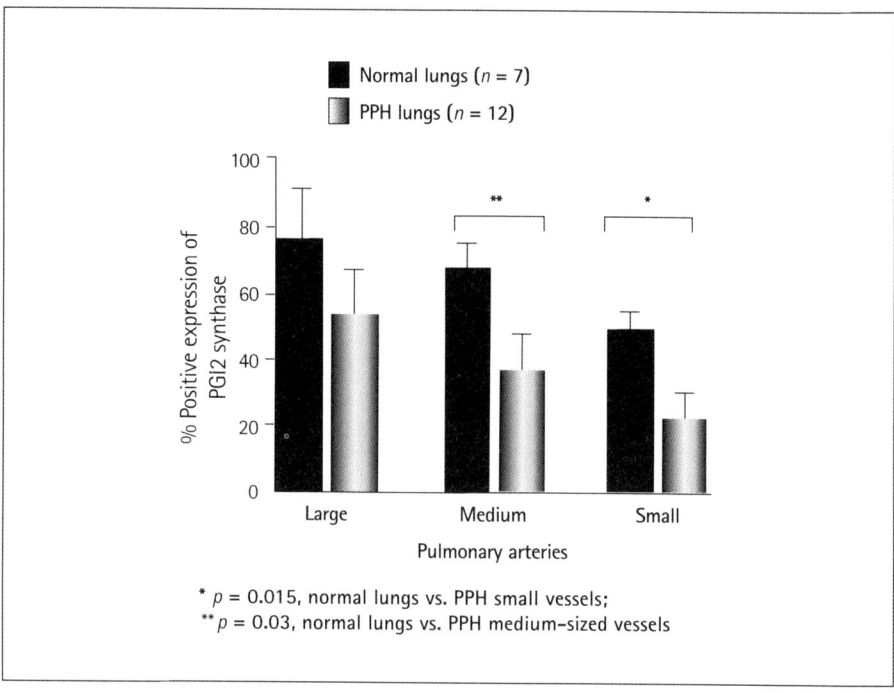

FIGURE 3   Evidence for reduction of prostacyclin synthase in the lungs of patients with severe pulmonary hypertension (PPH)[4]

platelet aggregation. These properties seemed very appropriate for the chronic treatment of patients with PPH, where there is a reduction of cardiac output and evidence of intravascular thrombosis.

PROSTANOID THERAPY: BENEFITS AND PROBLEMS

The disadvantage of prostacyclin pharmacologically is that it is rapidly hydrolyzed in the circulation and thereby inactivated; its double-ring structure is opened up as soon as the molecule comes into contact with oxygenated biological fluids. Consequently, prostacyclin has to be continuously delivered intravenously using a technically demanding system. Despite these practical problems of delivering the drug, the clinical outcome vindicated the rationale of its use; there was a phenomenal fall in pulmonary vascular resistance in our first case, which was be sustained for 2 years, allowing the patient to undergo lung transplantation (Figure 5)[1]. The first detailed randomized controlled trial showed a dramatic increase in walking distance, compared with a fall in the conventionally treated group[7] (Figure 6). More importantly, in a follow-on study, a dramatic increase in survival in people treated with prostacyclin was demonstrated, compared with historical controls[6].

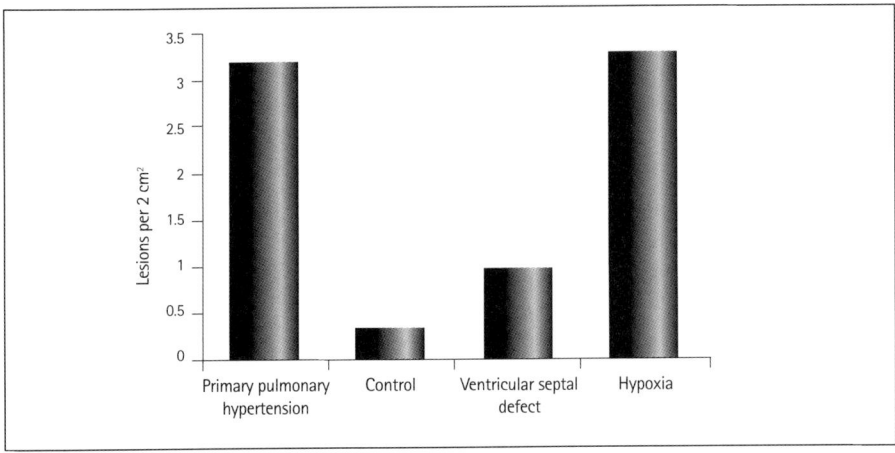

FIGURE 4   Density of intravascular thrombotic lesions in precapillary arteries of patients with pulmonary hypertension and other conditions, compared with controls[5]

TABLE 1   Primary pulmonary hypertension: cause of death. Data from the NIH Registry on PPH, 1991

Progressive right heart failure	47%
Sudden cardiac death	26%*
Other	26%

*Sudden cardiac death seen in NYHA Class IV patients

It seemed clear from all these studies that the vasodilatory and antithrombotic effects of prostacyclin were having sustained effects on the pulmonary circulation. There was, however, a problem, as prostacyclin seemed principally to be of benefit to those patients with the lowest cardiac index and the lowest mixed venous saturation, in other words, those in NYHA functional classes III–IV. It had no effect on survival in the earlier stages of disease. The other feature was that the benefit was not predictable from acute vasodilator responses at diagnostic right-heart catheterization, i.e. this was an accumulative effect of chronic treatment[8] (Table 3). In support of this was the study of McLaughlin and colleagues[9], which showed that, at 36 months, pulmonary vascular resistance had fallen below the level achieved with a maximum acute vasodilator test (adenosine), introducing the possibility of reversal of the pathology (Figure 7).

TABLE 2   The major prognostic measurements in primary pulmonary hypertension

Cardiac index
  Right atrial pressure
  Mixed venous oxygen saturation
  Pulmonary artery pressure

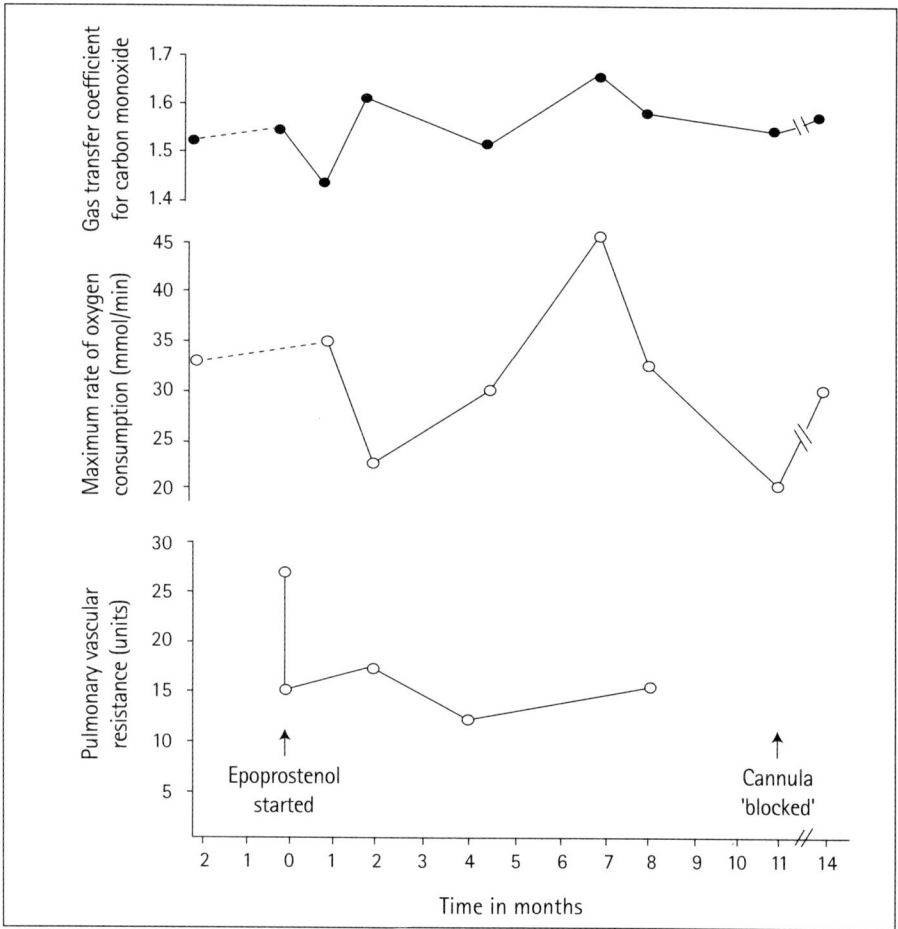

FIGURE 5   Positive effects of long-term prostanoid therapy of pulmonary hypertension[1]

WHO CLASSIFICATION OF PULMONARY HYPERTENSION

The demonstration that PGI2 improved survival in PPH led to attempts to use it in other forms of pulmonary hypertension. Not all attempts were successful. As a result, a new class-ification for pulmonary hypertension was sought (Figure 8). Largely at the instigation of

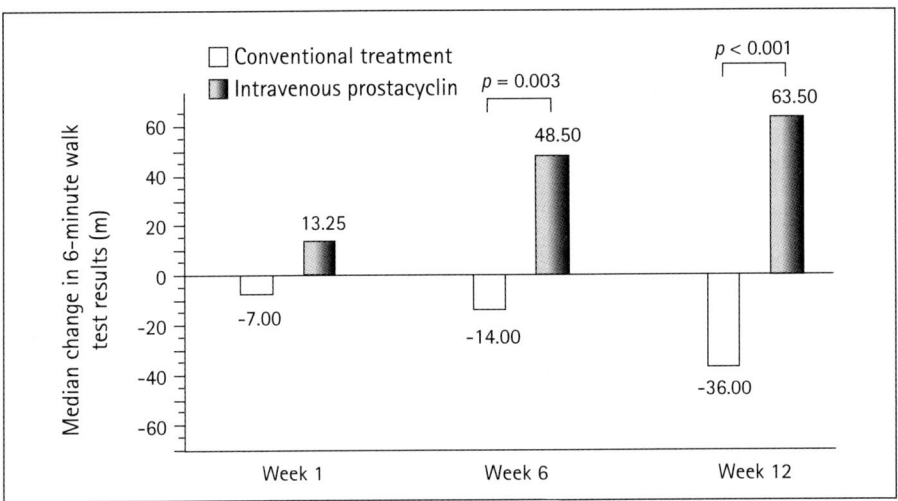

FIGURE 6   Improvement in exercise capacity in patients with pulmonary hypertension treated in a randomized controlled trial with intravenous prostacyclin[7]

TABLE 3   Prostaglandins and survival. Data from reference 8

	Patient survival			
	$SvO_2 > 63\%$		$SvO_2 < 63\%$	
	CT ($n = 28$)	PGI2 ($n = 16$)	CT ($n = 29$)	PGI2 ($n = 53$)
Median survival (days)	941	986	261	693*
Range (days)	427–2290	695–1590	42–612	326–1283

CT, right heart catheterization; SvO_2, venous oxygen saturation

Dr Stuart Rich, the World Health Organization (WHO) sponsored a meeting in 1998 to re-examine the classification of pulmonary hypertension. This meeting led to a scheme based upon anatomy but also upon the efficacy of the prostanoids in treating the different forms of the disease.

Five classes of pulmonary hypertension were selected at the WHO symposium. Pulmonary arterial hypertension was defined by the localization of the vascular narrowing in the pulmonary arteries, predominantly the small pre-capillary resistance vessels. Primary pulmonary hypertension, either sporadic or familial, is the most typical form of pulmonary arterial hypertension. These two disorders respond to intravenous prostanoids. Pulmonary arterial hypertension is found predominantly in patients with the associated diseases of scleroderma, portal hypertension, HIV infection and congenital heart disease. In all these

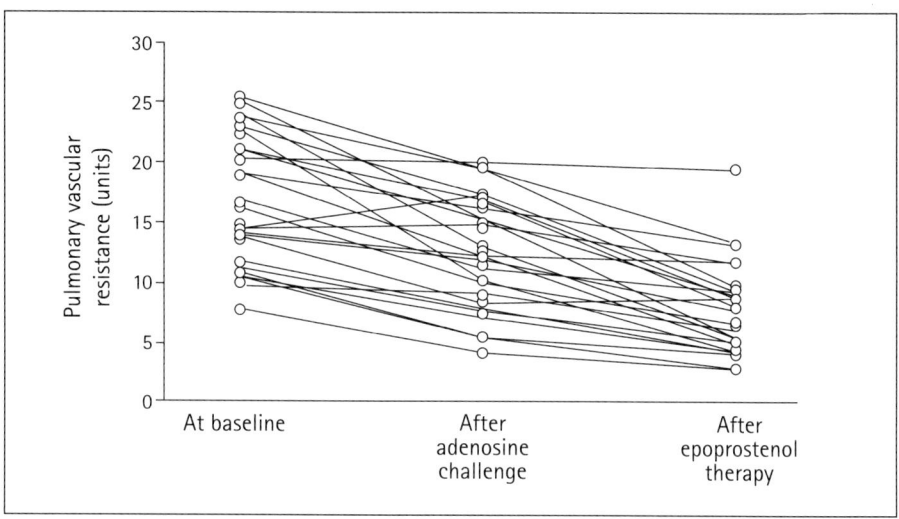

FIGURE 7   Progressive decline in pulmonary vascular resistance in patients with pulmonary hypertension treated with intravenous epoprostenol suggests the possibility of prostanoid therapy 'reversing' primary pulmonary hypertension[9]

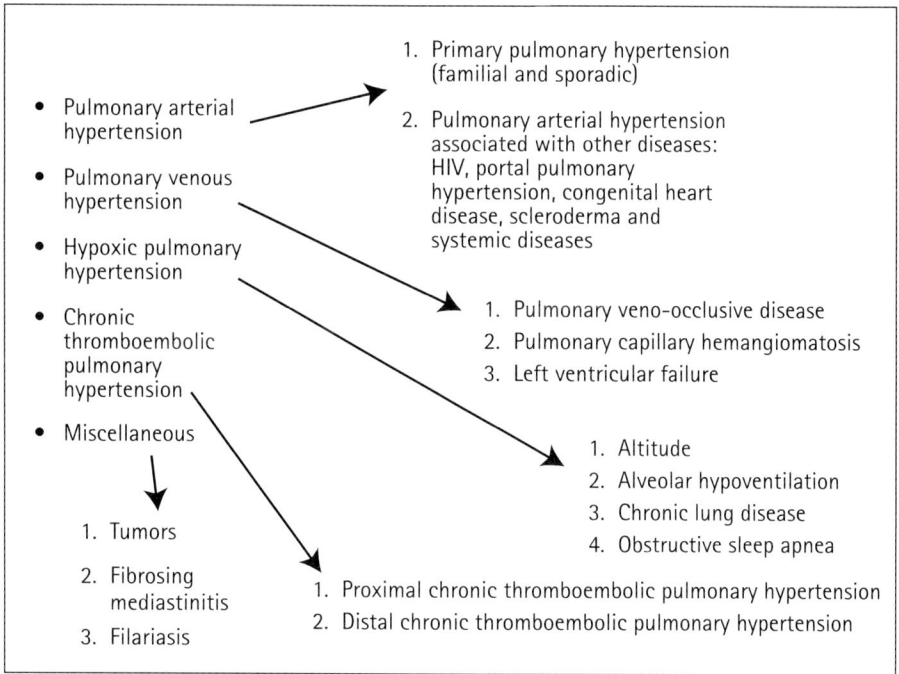

FIGURE 8   WHO classification of pulmonary hypertension, 1998

forms of pulmonary hypertension, intravenous prostanoids improve survival and exercise tolerance.

The next class is pulmonary venous hypertension in which the vascular narrowing is localized to veins. The most common forms are secondary to left ventricular failure and left-sided valvular disease. Intravenous prostanoid therapy in these forms of pulmonary hypertension worsens survival chances. Adverse effects with prostanoids are seen in the more unexplained forms of pulmonary venous hypertension, pulmonary veno-occlusive disease and pulmonary capillary hemangiomatosis.

In the third class of pulmonary hypertension, hypoxia, either as a consequence of lung disease or underventilation as in sleep apnea, there is widespread arterial narrowing and obstruction. Here, the general vasodilator effect of intravenous prostanoids may have a deleterious effect by increasing pulmonary shunt. Dilating vessels to poorly ventilated areas, constricted by hypoxia, will cause ventilation–perfusion mismatch, reducing effective gas exchange. This resultant fall in oxygen tension precludes the use of this therapy in this class of pulmonary hypertension.

The fourth class of pulmonary hypertension is a result of chronic thromboembolic disease. This is subdivided into a group with radiologically demonstrated proximal pulmonary artery obstruction and those without, where both show ventilation–perfusion mismatch on radionucleide imaging of the lung. Patients with proximal obstructions may respond favorably with surgical endarterectomy. Those patients considered suitable for surgery can be effectively treated with intravenous prostanoids.

The final class of pulmonary hypertension is made up of miscellaneous diseases including pulmonary artery sarcomas, mediastinal fibrosis and schistosomiasis. There is no information as to how these diseases are affected by prostanoids.

INHALED PROSTANOID THERAPY: THE NEXT STEP?

It should be possible to deliver prostanoids by alternative routes to the current complex delivery systems. One alternative is the inhaled route. This will be discussed in detail in Chapters 5 and 6. It has, however, been shown that, in PPH patients, aerosolized prostacyclin produces a very similar result to inhaled nitric oxide. In so doing it behaves as a selective pulmonary vasodilator. Furthermore, chronic treatment with aerosolized iloprost shows the long-term effectiveness seen with intravenous prostacyclin.

REFERENCES

1. Higenbottam T, Wheeldon D, Wells F, Wallwork, J. Long-term treatment of primary pulmonary hypertension with continuous intravenous epoprostenol (prostacyclin). *Lancet* 1984;1:1046–7

2. Rubin LJ, Groves BM, Reeves JT, Frosolono M, Handel F, Cato AE. Prostacyclin-induced acute pulmonary vasodilation in primary pulmonary hypertension. *Circulation* 1982;66:334–8

3. Fuster V, Steele PM, Edwards WD, Gersh BJ, McGoon MD, Frye RL. Primary pulmonary hypertension: natural history and the importance of thrombosis. *Circulation* 1984;70:580–7

4. Tuder R, Cool C, Geraci M, *et al.* Prostacyclin synthase expression is decreased in lungs from patients with severe pulmonary hypertension. *Am J Respir Crit Care Med* 1999;159:1925–32

5. Wagenvoort CA, Mulder PG. Thrombotic lesions in primary plexogenic arteriopathy. Similar pathogenesis or complication? *Chest* 1993;103:844–9

6. D'Alonzo GE, Barst RJ, Ayres SM, *et al.* (1991). Survival in patients with primary pulmonary hypertension. Results from a national prospective registry. *Ann Intern Med* 1991;115:343–9

7. Barst RJ, Rubin LJ, Long WA, *et al.* A comparison of continuous intravenous epoprostenol (prostacyclin) with conventional therapy for primary pulmonary hypertension. The Primary Pulmonary Hypertension Study Group. *N Engl J Med* 1996;334:296–302

8. Higenbottam T, Butt AY, McMahon A, Westerbeck R, Sharples L. Long-term intravenous prostaglandin (epoprostenol or iloprost) for treatment of severe pulmonary hypertension. *Heart* 1998;80:151–5

9. McLaughlin VV, Genthner DE, Panella MM, Rich S. Reduction in pulmonary vascular resistance with long-term epoprostenol (prostacyclin) therapy in primary pulmonary hypertension. *N Engl J Med* 1998;338:273–7

2

Pathophysiology of pulmonary arterial hypertension

R. Naeije

INTRODUCTION

Primary pulmonary hypertension (PPH) is a syndrome of dyspnea, fatigue, chest pain and syncope defined by an increase in pulmonary artery pressures and the absence of a known cause[1]. In the majority of patients, the condition is believed to evolve over years, with initially an asymptomatic increase in pulmonary arteriolar reactivity and remodelling. Signs and symptoms appear when mean pulmonay artery pressures are in the range of 30–40 mmHg at rest (normal pressure is < 20 mmHg). There is a progressive clinical deterioration when mean pulmonary artery pressures plateau around 60–70 mmHg and cardiac output progressively declines.

Pulmonary hypertension, that is indistinguishable from PPH in clinical course, histopathology and response to treatment, occurs in association with collagen vascular disease or congenital left-to-right shunting, and may be triggered by intake of appetite suppressants (mainly fenfluramines and aminorex), hypoxia, HIV infection or portal hypertension. Therefore, a recent consensus conference sponsored by the World Health Organization has proposed an extension of the concept of PPH to include these associated conditions, and to rename it 'pulmonary arterial hypertension' (PAH)[2]. The pathophysiology of PAH remains incompletely understood. Biological abnormalities of each compartment of the pulmonary vessel walls have been reported in patients with PAH.

GENETICS

In at least 6% of cases, PPH shows an autosomal dominant pattern of inheritance with reduced penetrance[1]. The gene for familial PPH (PPH1) has been mapped to chromosome 2q31–32[3]. There has been, until now, no heterogeneity, in other words no familial case has been found not to be linked to the *PPH1* gene. Recently, two different groups have reported a mutation in the *PPH1* gene which encodes bone morphogenetic protein receptor II (*BMPR2*), in nine of 19 families[4] and seven of eight families[5], respectively. The reported mutations are heterogeneous, and are believed to result in haplo-insufficiency, that is loss of function of one copy of the gene. Co-ancestry of *BMPR2* mutations has been shown in several cases of apparently sporadic PPH, suggesting that familial PPH may be more frequent than previously assumed[6]. However, carriers of *BMPR2* mutations have no more than 10–20% likelihood of developing clinically overt PPH[6], not all familial cases have detectable *BMPR2* mutations[4,5], and the incidence of *BMPR2* mutations does not seem to exceed 26% in sporadic PPH[7]. Mutations in another gene, *ALK1*, cause hereditary hemor-rhagic telangiectasia and, in at least some carriers, pulmonary vascular changes identical to those seen in PPH[8]. *ALK1* encodes the activin-receptor-like kinase 1, a TGF-β receptor, and pathogenic mutations are believed to result in haplo-insufficiency.

Bone morphogenetic proteins are members of the TGF-β superfamily of circulating proteins that regulate growth and repair of tissues in all organs[9]. Activation of TGF-βs can result in either promotion or inhibition of growth, depending on the cell and the circumstances[10]. While it appears likely that BMPRs, and other TGF-βs could play an important role in the control of vascular smooth muscle cell proliferation and apoptosis, at this stage it is not at all clear exactly how[10]. The observation, that mutations in two different, but mechanisti-cally related, TGF-β receptors can produce the same clinical phenotype, suggests interaction to modulate vascular growth, but again by yet unknown cellular mechanisms. It is possible that *BMPR2* mutations would be involved mainly in smooth muscle cell proliferation, and *ALK1* mutations in endothelial cell proliferation[10]. Since *BMPR2* and *ALK1* mutations are neither a necessary nor a sufficient cause for PPH, it is speculated that gene modifiers such as environmental factors, estrogens, or additional mutations in unknown regulatory genes may be required for the clinical expression of the disease[10]. Further experimental testing will be needed to identify *BMPR2* and *ALK1* gene modifiers and their mode of action. Improved knowledge of the function of *BMPR2* and *ALK1* will also help us to understand why the genetic defect, which is present from birth and affects a wide range of tissues, leads to disease that is restricted to the pulmonary circulation, and becomes manifest relatively late in life. It will also be interesting to establish the exact incidence of *ALK1* and *BMPR2* mutations in non-strictly primary PAH subcategories.

PLEXIFORM LESIONS

Many patients with PPH present with a peculiar pulmonary vascular focal structure, the plexiform lesion, the features of which include obstruction of the arterial lumen, aneurysmal dilatation, proliferation of interconnected vascular channels, and endothelial and smooth muscle cell proliferations[11,12]. Plexiform lesions are found in about one- to two-thirds of pathologic examinations of lung tissue specimens from PPH patients[11,12]. However, plexiform lesions are not specific for PPH, as they are also observed in patients with pulmonary hypertension secondary to congenital heart disease[11] and scleroderma[13].

Plexiform lesions are generally believed to result from an angiogenic response to local ischemia or hypoxia, occurring distal to vascular obstructive lesions. It has been suggested that plexiform lesions may represent a tumor-like proliferation of endothelial cells, possibly triggered by pulmonary vascular inflammation and/or cell death[13]. The proliferation of endothelial cells in plexiform lesions has been shown to be monoclonal in PPH, but polyclonal in secondary pulmonary hypertension[14]. There has been speculation that dysregulated endothelial cell growth could be related to *BMPR* mutations[15]. However, the notion of PPH being a particular type of endothelial cell cancer does not fit with the most early stages of the disease, characterized by medial hypertrophy rather than by plexiform lesions[1,11,12], and with the observation of a similar clinical course, histopathology and response to prostacyclin therapy of pulmonary hypertension, with either monoclonal or polyclonal endothelial cell proliferation in plexiform lesions, or even without any plexiform lesions.

INFLAMMATION

Areas of focal necrosis with inflammatory reactions have long been described in the walls of pulmonary vessels of patients with PAH[11,12]. More recently, perivascular inflammatory cell infiltrates, with T and B lymphocytes and macrophages, were shown to occur in plexiform lesions of patients with PAH[13]. Increased circulating levels of the pro-inflammatory cytokines, interleukin-1β and interleukin-6, which both promote thrombosis and are potent mitogens, have been measured in patients with PPH[16]. Platelet-derived growth factor expression is elevated in lung biopsies from PPH patients[17]. Perivascular inflammatory or even intravascular inflammatory cell accumulation may be the source of a series of growth factors and cytokines contributing to vessel wall remodelling and *in situ* microthrombosis.

COAGULATION

Patients with PAH present with decreased platelet count and enhanced platelet activity, with increased circulating levels of serotonin, plasminogen activator inhibitor, and fibrinopeptide A, and decreased thrombomodulin levels[18]. Thrombotic lesions are identified in about one-third of PPH patients[11,12]. Anticoagulant therapy improves survival in patients with PPH[19]. It is thus likely that hypercoagulability and *in situ* microthrombosis contribute to the progression of the disease, if not to its initiation. The role of abnormal coagulation in subcategories of PAH that are not strictly primary is less well established.

SEROTONIN AND THE SEROTONIN TRANSPORTER

A series of observations suggest that serotonin is a potential trigger/perpetrator of PAH. Patients with PPH have increased levels of circulating serotonin and decreased platelet serotonin concentrations, and these abnormalities persist after heart–lung transplantation[20]. Intake of fenfluramines was associated with an epidemic of PPH in France and in Belgium in the early 1990s[21,22]. These drugs induce the release and inhibit the reuptake of serotonin by platelets and nerve endings. Fawn-hooded rats, which have an inherited platelet storage defect, develop pulmonary hypertension when bred in even a mildly hypoxic environment, and with aging[23]. Low-dose intravenous serotonin, titrated to reproduce plasma levels measured in patients treated with fenfluramines, enhances hypoxic pulmonary vasoconstriction and chronic hypoxia-induced pulmonary vascular remodelling in the rat[24]. In dogs, dexfenfluramine has been shown to enhance hypoxic pulmonary vasoconstriction after acute intravenous administration[25], and to increase pulmonary vascular resistance by about 25% after chronic oral intake for 20 days[26]. Thus naturally or drug-induced increases in circulating serotonin may be involved in the pathogenesis of PAH.

However, the mechanisms of serotonin-induced pulmonary vasoreactivity and remodelling remain unclear. The mitogenic effects of serotonin on pulmonary artery smooth muscle cells require the expression of a serotonin transporter, which is inhibited by fenfluramines but promoted by discontinuation of fenfluramine therapy[27]. Mice lacking the 5-hydroxytryptamine transporter gene are relatively protected against pulmonary vascular remodelling and hypertension in chronically hypoxic conditions[28]. The ability to inhibit the serotonin transporter is shared by serotoninergic antidepressant drugs such as fluoxetine and paroxetine. Serotoninergic antidepressant drugs may have a more persistent inhibitor effect on the serotonin transporter, as their chronic intake seems to be associated with a decreased, instead of an increased, risk of developing PAH[29]. Recent studies have shown that serotonin transporter overexpression is responsible for pulmonary artery smooth muscle hyperplasia in PPH[30]. At this stage, there may be sufficient evidence to support a clinical trial of serotonin transporter inhibitor, for example with antidepressant drugs, in patients with PAH.

ENDOTHELIUM

Pulmonary vascular tone is modulated by balanced actions of endothelium-derived vasodilators, mainly prostacyclin and nitric oxide (NO), and vasodilators, mainly thromboxane A2 and endothelin. Patients with PAH present with an increased 24-h urinary excretion of thromboxane B2, the stable metabolite of thromboxane A2, and a decreased 24-h urinary excretion of 6-keto-$PGF_{1\alpha}$, the stable metabolite of prostacyclin[31]. Pulmonary arterial endothelial cells of PAH patients present with an increased expression of endothelin synthase[32] and reduced expressions of NO synthase[33] and prostacyclin synthase[34]. Endothelin levels are increased in patients with PAH[35]. Chronic treatment with prostacyclin derivatives, given intravenously[36], subcutaneously[37], by inhalation[38], or even orally[39] improves clinical state, functional class, exercise capacity and survival in patients with PAH. Beneficial effects have also been reported with chronic treatment with bosentan, an oral endothelin receptor antagonist, in patients with PPH or with scleroderma-associated PAH[40]. Chronic inhaled NO has been used in some patients with severe pulmonary hypertension as a bridge to heart–lung transplantation[41]. While none of these treatments offers a cure, their efficacy is in keeping with the notion that an endothelial-derived vasoconstrictor–vasodilator imbalance plays a significant role in the progression of PAH.

PULMONARY ARTERY SMOOTH MUSCLE

Studies on freshly dispersed isolated pulmonary artery smooth muscle cells have shown that acute hypoxia inhibits a potassium current, causing membrane depolarization and secondary entry of calcium, leading to vasoconstriction and possibly initiating cell proliferation[42]. The potassium channels inhibited by hypoxia belong to the voltage-gated type (Kv), and have been identified in pulmonary artery smooth muscle cells of rats as $Kv_{1.5}$ and $Kv_{2.1}$[43]. Isolated pulmonary artery smooth muscle cells of patients with PPH present with decreased $Kv_{1.5}$ mRNA levels[44]. The $Kv_{2.1}$ channel is inhibited by the appetite suppressant drugs aminorex and dexfenfluramine[45]. These observations support the idea of a unique mechanism accounting for enhanced pulmonary vasoreactivity and subsequent remodelling in hypoxic pulmonary hypertension, as well as in the various PAH subcategories, and confirm the chronically hypoxic rodent as a valid experimental PAH model. However, more experimental data appear to be needed to define the role of abnormal voltage-gated potassium channel function in PAH. Recently, a series of serotoninergic mood-enhancing and/or appetite-decreasing drugs, aminorex, phentermine, dexfenfluramine, sibutramine, and fluoxetine, were shown to inhibit a cloned $Kv_{1.5}$ channel stably expressed in a mammalian cell line[46]. In that study, the most potent inhibitors of the $Kv_{1.5}$ channel were sibutramine and fluoxetine, which have not been associated with an increased incidence of PAH[46]. Further research is needed to determine whether abnormal voltage-gated potassium channels could be a cause or a response in PAH, and which specific potassium channel might be involved.

ADVENTITIUM

Vascular remodelling is a prominent feature in PAH. Pulmonary vessels of patients with PAH show variable combinations of intimal fibrosis, medial hypertrophy and extension, but also advential changes with increased extracellular matrix production[2]. It has been suggested that endothelial abnormalities early in the course of PAH allow for the extravasation of factors that stimulate smooth muscle cells to produce a vascular serine elastase[47]. This results in the liberation of matrix-bound smooth muscle cell mitogens, such as basic fibrobast growth factor, and enhances matrix degradation by activating other matrix metalloproteases (MMP). The MMPs can stimulate the production of tenascin, a mitogenic cofactor which produces phosphorylation of growth factor receptors and smooth muscle cell proliferation[47]. Monocrotaline-induced pulmonary hypertension in rats can indeed be completely reversed by a serine elastase inhibitor[48]. However, inhibition of MMP by lung transfer metalloprotease-1 or by the administration of doxycycline aggravates chronic hypoxia-induced pulmonary hypertension in rats[49]. Thus, while these observations are in keeping with the notion that all three layers of the pulmonary arterial wall interact to trigger and perpetuate PAH, it is not presently clear, on the basis of experimental animal observations, exactly which adventitial dysfunction could be targeted by future therapeutic interventions in humans.

CONCLUSIONS

Recent years have witnessed important advances in knowledge of the pathophysiological understanding of PAH. Although the initial event leading to the onset of a progressive increase in PVR remains unknown, several important mechanisms that concur to perpetrate the disease process have now been identified, and pharmacological manipulation of some of them has already proved clinically beneficial. At present, manipulation of disrupted equilibrium between endothelium-derived vasoconstrictors and vasodilators remains the best established therapeutic option, but new approaches aimed at the correction of medial and adventitial abnormalities are soon likely to be evaluated in clinical trials. A multi-drug approach might offer the perspective of halting or even reversing the progression of PAH in the near future.

REFERENCES

1. Rubin LJ. Primary pulmonary hypertension. *N Engl J Med* 1997;33:111–17

2. Rich S, ed. *Primary pulmonary hypertension: executive summary from the World Symposium on Primary Pulmonary Hypertension 1998.* Geneva: World Health Organization, 1998 (http//www.who.int/ncd/cvd/pph.html)

3. Nichols WC, Koller DL, Slovis B, *et al.* Localisation of the gene for familial primary pulmonary hypertension to chromosome 2q31-32. *Nat Genet* 1997;15:277–80

4. Deng Z, Morse JH, Slager SL, *et al.* Familial primary pulmonary hypertension gene PPH1 is caused by mutations in bone morphogenetic protein receptor-II gene. *Am J Hum Genet* 2000;67:737–44

5. The International PPH Consortium. Heterozygous germline mutations in BMPR2, encoding a TGF-β receptor, cause familial primary pulmonary hypertension. *Nat Genet* 2000;26:81–4

6. Newman JH, Wheeler L, Lane KB, *et al.* Mutation in the gene for bone morphogenetic protein receptor II as a cause of pulmonary hypertension in a large kindred. *N Engl J Med* 2001;345:319–24

7. Thomson JR, Machado RD, Panciulo MW, *et al.* Sporadic primary pulmonary hypertension is associated with germline mutations of the gene encoding for BMPR-II, a receptor of the TGF-beta family. *J Med Genet* 2000;37:741–5

8. Trembath RC, Thomson JR, Machado RD, *et al.* Clinical and molecular genetic features of pulmonary hypertension in patients with hereditary hemorrhagic telangiectasia. *N Engl J Med* 2001;345:325–34

9. Massague J, Blain SW, Lo RS. TGF-beta signalling in growth control, cancer, and inheritable disorders. *Cell* 2000;103:295–309

10. Loscalzo J. Genetic clues to the cause of primary pulmonary hypertension. *N Engl J Med* 2001;345:367–70

11. Wagenvoort CA, Wagenvoort N. Primary pulmonary hypertension : a pathological study of the lung vessels in 156 clinically diagnosed cases. *Circulation* 1970;42:1163–84

12. Pietra GG, Edwards WD, Kay M, *et al.* Histopathology of primary pulmonary hypertension: a qualitative and quantitative study of pulmonary blood vessels from 58 patients in the National Heart, Lung and Blood Institute, Primary Pulmonary Hypertension Registry. *Circulation* 1989;80:1207–21

13. Tuder RM, Groves BM, Badesch DB, Voelkel NF. Exuberant endothelial cell growth and elements of inflammation are present in plexiform lesions of pulmonary hypertension. *Am J Pathol* 1994;144:275–85

14. Lee SD, Shroyer KR, Markham NE, Cool CD, Voelkel NF, Tuder RM. Monoclonal endothelial cell proliferation is present in primary but not secondary pulmonary hypertension. *J Clin Invest* 1998;101:927–34

15. Tuder RM, Yeager ME, Geraci M, Golpon HA, Voelkel NF. Severe pulmonary hypertension after the discovery of the familial primary pulmonary hypertension gene. *Eur Respir J* 2001;17:1065–9

16. Humbert M, Monti G, Brenot F, *et al.* Increased interleukin-1 and interleukin-6 serum concentrations in severe pulmonary hypertension. *Am J Respir Crit Care Med* 1995;151:1628–31

17. Humbert M, Monti G, Fartoukh M, *et al.* Platelet-derived growth factor expression in primary pulmonary hypertension : comparison of HIV seropositive and HIV seronegative patients. *Eur Respir J* 1998;11:554–9

18. Welsh CH, Hassell KL, Badesch DB, *et al.* Coagulation and fibrinolytic profiles in patients with severe pulmonary hypertension. *Chest* 1996;110:710–17

19. Fuster V, Steele PM, Edwards WD, *et al.* Primary pulmonary hypertension : natural history and importance of thrombosis. *Circulation* 1984;70:580–7

20. Hervé P, Launay JM, Scrobohaci ML, *et al.* Increased plasma serotonin in primary pulmonary hypertension. *Am J Med* 1995;99:249–54

21. Abenhaim L, Moride Y, Brenot F, *et al.* Appetite-suppressant drugs and the risk of primary pulmonary hypertension. *N Engl J Med* 1996;335:609–16

22. Delcroix M, Kurtz X, Walckiers D, Demedts M, Naeije R. High incidence of primary pulmonary hypertension associated with appetite suppressants in Belgium. *Eur Respir J* 1998;12:271–6

23. Sato K, Webb S, Tucker A, *et al*. Factors influencing the idiopathic development of pulmonary hypertension in the fawn-hooded rat. *Am Rev Respir Dis* 1992;145:793–7

24. Eddahibi S, Raffestin B, Pham I, *et al*. Treatment with 5-HT potentiates development of pulmonary hypertension in chronically hypoxic rats. *Am J Physiol* 1997;272(Heart Circ Physiol 41):H1173–81

25. Naeije R, Wauthy P, Maggiorini M, Leeman M, Delcroix M. Effects of dexfenfluramine on hypoxic pulmonary vasoconstriction and on embolic pulmonary hypertension in dogs. *Am J Respir Crit Care Med* 1995;151:642–7

26. Naeije R, Maggiorini M, Delcroix M, Leeman M, Mélot M. Effects of chronic dexfenfluramine treatment on pulmonary hemodynamics in dogs. *Am J Respir Crit Care Med* 1996;154:1347–51

27. Eddahibi S, Adnot S, Frisdal E, *et al*. Dexfenfluramine-associated changes in 5-hydroxy-tryptamine transporter expression and development of hypoxic pulmonary hypertension in rats. *J Pharmacol Ther* 2001;297:148–54

28. Eddahibi S, Hanoun N, Lanfumey L, *et al*. Attenuated hypoxic pulmonary hypertension in mice lacking the 5-hydroxytryptamine transporter gene. *J Clin Invest* 2000;105:1555–62

29. Abenhaim L, Rich S, Benichou J, Begaud B. Primary pulmonary hypertension and anorectic drugs. *N Engl J Med* 1999;340:482–3

30. Eddahibi S, Humbert M, Fadel E, *et al*. Serotonin transporter overexpression is responsible for pulmonary artery smooth muscle hyperplasia in primary pulmonary hypertension. *J Clin Invest* 2001;108:1141–50

31. Christman BW, McPherson CD, Newman JH, *et al*. An imbalance between the excretion of thromboxane and prostacyclin metabolites in pulmonary hypertension. *N Engl J Med* 1992;327:70–5

32. Giaid A, Salch D. Reduced expression of endothelial nitric oxide synthase in the lungs of patients with pulmonary hypertension. *N Engl J Med* 1995;333:214–21

33. Giaid A, Yamagisawa M, Langleben D, Michel RP, Levy R, Shennib H. Expression of endothe-lin-1 in the lungs of patients with pulmonary hypertension. *N Engl J Med* 1993;328:1732–9

34. Tuder RM, Cool CD, Geraci MW, *et al*. Prostacyclin synthase expression is decreased in lungs from patients with severe pulmonary hypertension. *Am J Respir Crit Care Med* 1999;159:1925–32

35. Cacoub P, Dorent R, Maistre G, *et al.* Endothelin-1 in primary pulmonary hypertension and the Eisenmenger syndrome. *Am J Cardiol* 1993;71:448–50

36. Barst, RJ, Rubin LJ, Long WA, *et al.* A comparison of continuous intravenous epoprostenol (prostacyclin) with conventional therapy for primary pulmonary hypertension. *N Engl J Med* 1996;334:296–301

37. Barst R, Simonneau G, Rich S, Blackburn S, Naeije R, Rubin LJ. Efficacy and safety of chronic subcutaneous infusion of UT-15 in pulmonary arterial hypertension. *Circulation* 2000;102(Suppl):100

38. Hoeper MM, Schwarze M, Ehlerding S, *et al.* Long-term treatment of primary pulmonary hypertension with aerosolized iloprost, a prostacyclin analogue. *N Engl J Med* 2000;342:1866–70

39. Nagaya N, Uematsu M, Okano Y, *et al.* Effect of orally active prostacyclin analogue on survival of outpatients with primary pulmonary hypertension. *J Am Coll Cardiol* 1999;34:1188–92

40. Channick R, Badesch DB, Tapson VF, *et al.* Effects of the dual endothelin receptor antagonist bosentan in patients with pulmonary hypertension: a placebo-controlled study. *J Heart Lung Transplant* 2001;20:262–3

41. Snell GI, Salamonsen RF, Begin P, *et al.* Inhaled nitric oxide as a bridge to heart–lung transplantation in a patient with end-stage pulmonary hypertension. *Am J Respir Crit Care Med* 1995;151:1263–6

42. Weir EK, Archer SL. The mechanisms of acute hypoxic pulmonary vasoconstriction: the tale of two channels. *FASEB J* 1995;9:183–9

43. Archer SL, Souil E, Dinh-Xuan AT, *et al.* Molecular identification of the role of voltage-gated K+ channels, Kv1.5 and Kv2.1, in hypoxic pulmonary vasoconstriction and control of resting membrane potential in rat pulmonary artery myocytes. *J Clin Invest* 1998;101:2319–30

44. Yuan XJ, Wang J, Juhuszova M, *et al.* Attenuated K+ channel gene transcription in primary pulmonary hypertension. *Lancet* 1998;351:726–7

45. Weir EK, Reeve HL, Huang JMC, *et al.* Anorectic agents aminorex, fenfluramine, and dexfenfluramine inhibit potassium current in rat pulmonary vascular smooth muscle and cause pulmonary vasoconstriction. *Circulation* 1996;94:2216–20

46. Perchenet L, Hilfiger L, Mizrahi J, Clement-Chomienne O. Effects of anorexinogen agents on cloned voltage-gated K(+) channel hKv1.5. *J Pharmacol Exp Ther* 2001;298:1108–19

47. Cowan KN, Jones PL, Rabinovitch M, *et al.* Elastase and matrix metalloproteinase inhibitors induce regression, and tenascin antisense prevents progression of vascular disease. *J Clin Invest* 2000;105:21–34

48. Cowan KN, Heilbut A, Humpl T, Lam C, Ito S, Rabinovitch M. Complete reversal of fatal pulmonary hypertension in rats by a serine elastase inhibitor. *Nat Med* 2000;6:698–702

49. Vieillard-Baron A, Frisdal E, Eddahibi S, *et al.* Inhibition of matrix metalloproteinases by lung TIMP-1 gene transfer or doxycycline aggravates pulmonary hypertension in rats. *Circ Res* 2000;87:418–25

Routes of administration of prostanoids

G. Simonneau

3

There is a great deal of evidence that low levels of prostacyclin, with associated dysregulation of metabolic pathways, play an important part in the pathophysiology of pulmonary arterial hypertension (PAH)[1,2]. Consequently, there is a strong rationale for the use of prostanoid therapy in the treatment of these patients. The administration of prostacyclin by continuous intravenous infusion is the only pharmacologic therapy approved for use in Europe and the USA for primary pulmonary hypertension (PPH), and also for patients with scleroderma PAH in New York Heart Association (NYHA) functional classes III or IV. This approval is based on two randomized, controlled, open-label trials, one carried out in PPH patients[3], which showed a beneficial effect on mortality, and the other, in scleroderma patients[4], which demonstrated improvements in exercise capacity and hemodynamic parameters. Despite the lack of randomized, controlled trials, many clinicians also acknowledge that calcium antagonists are probably very effective for the treatment of PAH, but only in a small minority of patients (<10%)[5].

Prostacyclin has a very short half-life of about 1–2 min and therefore has to be delivered by continuous intravenous infusion. Although intravenous prostacyclin therapy of PAH is very effective in terms of reduced mortality, it is a complicated treatment with some substantial disadvantages[6]. Persistent minor prostacyclin-related side-effects include headache, jaw pain, diarrhea, nausea and flushing. Severe complications include ascites and especially pulmonary edema, which affects a subgroup of patients with pulmonary veno-occlusive disease (PVO) and pulmonary capillary hemangiomatosis (PCH). However, the most frequent complications are a result of the need to use a central intravenous catheter delivery system, namely, infection, thrombosis, bleeding, and pneumothorax and rapid deterioration when the infusion is stopped. In our center, the infection rate associated with intravenous prostacyclin therapy is 0.5 per patient-year. Also, with long-term use of intravenous prostacyclin, patients develop tolerance (tachyphylaxis) and it is necessary to increase the dose, thus escalating the costs of treatment. In France, the annual cost of treating one patient with intravenous prostacyclin therapy for PAH is estimated at about 1 million French francs.

Several other modes of administration of prostanoids have been investigated that are less invasive, potentially less costly, and associated with fewer severe complications. They include continuous subcutaneous infusion, inhalation therapy (using six to nine inhalations per day), and oral therapy, currently using beraprost sodium and perhaps, in the near future, oral iloprost. The use of inhalation therapy with iloprost is considered in Chapters 5 and 6; the focus in this chapter will therefore be on the subcutaneous delivery of the stable prostacyclin analog treprostinol and oral therapy with beraprost sodium.

SUBCUTANEOUS TREPROSTINOL THERAPY

Unlike prostacyclin, treprostinol is chemically stable at room temperature and neutral pH and can be delivered by subcutaneous infusion. Hence, in contrast to prostacyclin therapy, there is no need to use a central intravenous catheter and there are, therefore, no risks of infection or thrombosis. In addition, there is no need to reconstitute the solution, no need for refrigeration, and, overall, a better patient compliance. Treprostinol is also less expensive than prostacyclin and its much longer half-life means that it carries no risks of a rapid deterioration in the condition of the patient if the infusion pump fails. Delivery of treprostinol uses a smaller infusion pump (MiniMed, United Therapeutics, USA) than that used for prostacyclin and has the additional advantage that the patient is him/herself able to insert the catheter into the tissue of the abdominal wall. Similarly, the catheter can be changed by the patient, as required, which is normally every 1–3 days.

The clinical evaluation of treprostinol has been carried out in a large randomized, double-blind study involving 470 patients recruited from centers in Europe and the USA (Table 1)[7]. Most of the patients entered into the study had a diagnosis of PPH, but others had connective tissue disorders or congenital heart disease with systemic-to-pulmonary shunts. About 80% of patients were in NYHA class III, with smaller numbers in classes II and IV. The primary endpoint of the study was the distance attained at week 12 in the 6-min walk test, the mean distance covered at baseline being 326 ± 6 m.

As prescribed in the trial protocol, the treprostinol dose was titrated to the maximum level consistent with acceptable side-effects or to the maximum allowed dose of 22 ng/kg/min.

As expected, the maximum dose achieved in the placebo group was considerably higher than that in the active treatment group (Table 2). The main side-effect observed was pain at the site of infusion, which occurred in virtually all patients; it required dose reductions in 23% of patients and permanent cessation of therapy in 8% (Table 3). Some patients experienced some very severe local reactions, often precluding a rapid increase in dose or requiring termination of treatment.

After 12 weeks' treprostinol therapy, the statistically adjusted distance attained in the 6-min walk test increased by 16 m, compared with no increase in the placebo group; this was

TABLE 1   Baseline characteristics of clinical evaluation of treprostinol in a randomized, double-blind study of patients with primary pulmonary hypertension (PPH) or collagen vascular disease[7] or congenital heart disease[7]. Data are given as mean ± standard error or percentage

	Treprostinol (n = 233)	Placebo (n = 236)
Age (years)	45 ± 1	44 ± 1
Gender (female)	85%	78%
PAH etiology		
PPH	58%	58%
CVD	17%	20%
CHD	25%	22%
NYHA		
class II	11%	12%
class III	82%	81%
class IV	8%	7%
Six-min walk (m)	326 ± 5	327 ± 6

PAH, pulmonary arterial hypertension; CVD, collagen vascular disease; CHD, congenital heart disease

TABLE 2   Maximum doses achieved in the treprostinol and placebo groups consistent with acceptable side-effects

	Dose (ng/kg/min)	
	Week 6	Week 12
Treprostinol	5.9 ± 0.21	9.3 ± 0.38
Placebo	10.0 ± 0.21	19.1 ± 0.33

highly significant ($p = 0.0064$; see Table 4), although the improvement was of minor clinical significance. Interestingly, there was a very close relationship between the treprostinol dose delivered and the outcome of the 6-min walk test, such that the improvement obtained at the highest delivered dose of 16.2 ng/kg/min was a very clinically significant 36 m, compared with no improvement with the 2.5 ng/kg/min dose (Figure 1). Also, improvements in the 6-min walk test correlated with baseline features that suggest that the therapy is more effective in severely ill patients with a low mixed oxygen venous saturation (SvO_2) and poor initial exercise capacity (Table 5).

A number of secondary endpoints were also measured in the study, including dyspnea, clinical symptoms and cardiopulmonary hemodynamic parameters; however, all improved with treprostinol therapy (no data presented). As regards patient outcome, the numbers of deaths were low in both groups and not significantly different; however, there were significant differences in the incidence of painful infusion sites (Table 6).

TABLE 3   Local reactions at site of infusion

	Treprostinol	Placebo
Overall incidence	234 (> 99%)	180 (> 77%)*
Requiring dose reduction	55 (23%)	2 (< 1%)*
Requiring temporary stopping	3 (1%)	0 (0%)
Requiring permanent stopping	18 (8%)	0 (0%)*

*$p < 0.05$

TABLE 4   Exercise capacity: 6-min walk

	Median change from baseline (m)		Distance in median distance walked (m)*	p Value
	Treprostinol	Placebo		
Week 12	+ 10	0	+ 16	0.0064
Week 6	+ 13	+ 4	+ 11	0.032
Week 1	+ 11	+ 8	+ 5	0.27

* Non-parametic analysis of covariance (Hodges–Lehmann estimate)

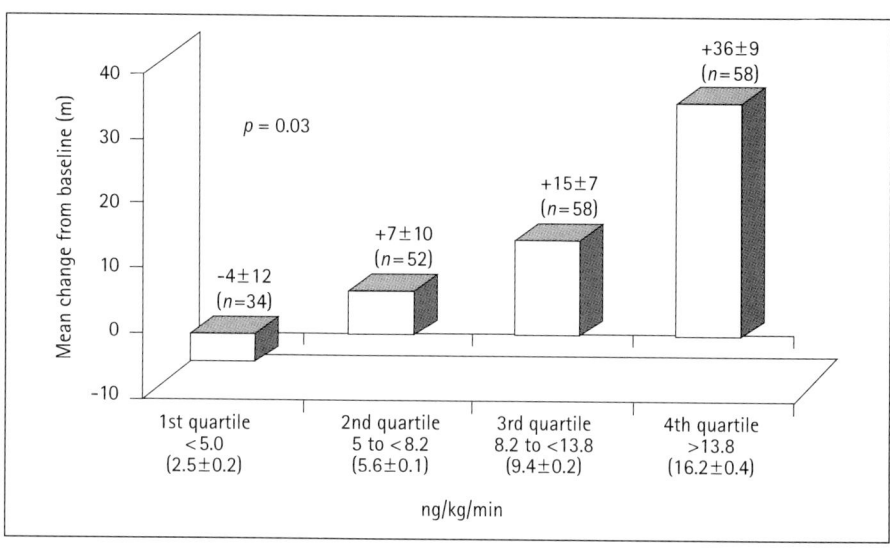

FIGURE 1   The effect of mean delivered dose of treprostinol on the change from baseline to week 12 in exercise capacity measured with the 6-min walk test[7]

TABLE 5   Treprostinol: predictors of change in the 6-min walk test

Covariate	p Value
Gender	0.4278
Race	0.8302
Age	0.3843
Etiology (PPH, CVD, CHD)	0.5985
NYHA classification	0.1051
Baseline walk	0.0338
SvO_2	0.0728
Vasodilator use at baseline	0.3427

PPH, primary pulmonary hypertension; CVD, collagen vascular disease; CHD, congenital heart disease; SvO_2, venous oxygen saturation

The treprostinol trial was the first double-blind, placebo-controlled study of PPH and other forms of PAH, and the largest study of severe pulmonary hypertension ever to have been carried out. It has shown some very positive findings, demonstrating the efficacy of treprostinol therapy in terms of the primary and secondary endpoints, without life-threatening side-effects. There were also some negative findings, including a lack of any effect on mortality, an improvement in exercise capacity that was statistically significant but was less than expected, and the almost universal occurrence of local infusion site reactions, precluding dose escalation in some patients and leading to premature discontinuation in 8%.

ORAL BERAPROST SODIUM

Beraprost is the first stable prostacyclin analog suitable for oral administration (Figure 2). It has a short half-life of only 36 min and requires to be taken at least four times daily. It has been evaluated in the ALPHABET trial[8], a European double-blind, randomized, controlled

TABLE 6   Patient outcome of treprostinol therapy for 12 weeks

	Treprostinol n (%)	Placebo n (%)
Completed 12 weeks	200 (86)	221 (93)
Treatment failures		
death	7 (3)	7 (3)
transplantation	0	1 (< 1)
deterioration	6 (3)	6 (3)
Withdrawal of consent	2 (1)	1 (< 1)
Adverse events	18 (8)	1 (< 1)

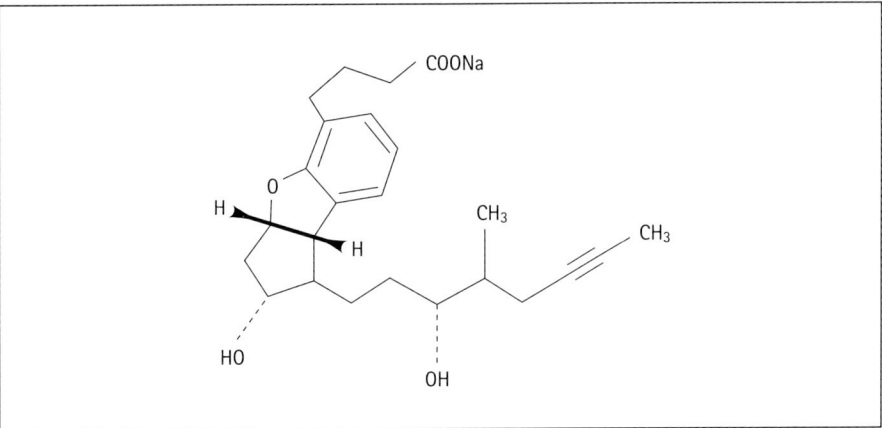

FIGURE 2   The chemical structure of beraprost sodium

study carried out in 130 patients in six countries, 65 receiving beraprost sodium and 65 given a placebo. A notable feature of the patients entered into the trial (Table 7) is that only 48% had PPH, the remainder having secondary pulmonary hypertension due to a number of diverse conditions, namely, congenital cardiac shunt, portal hypertension, collagen vascular disease, and HIV infection. It is noteworthy that the trial was also the first to include patients from NYHA class II, which constituted about half of those entered (Table 7). The patients in the study had severe pulmonary hypertension with markedly elevated pulmonary arterial pressure (PAP) and a low cardiac index (CI). In comparison with the treprostinol trial reviewed above, patients in the beraprost study had a greater baseline exercise capacity, as reflected in the mean distance attained in the 6-min walk test of 362 ± 94 m.

TABLE 7 Baseline characteristics of the patients entered into the ALPHABET trial of beraprost sodium versus placebo therapy[8]. Data are given as mean $\pm$ standard deviation or number (percentage)

	Beraprost sodium ($n = 65$)	Placebo ($n = 65$)
Age (years)	46 ± 16	45 ± 14
Gender		
female	42 (65%)	38 (59%)
male	23 (35%)	27 (41%)
PPH	35 (54%)	28 (43%)
Etiology		
congenital cardiac shunt	9 (14%)	15 (23%)
portal hypertension	12 (18%)	9 (14%)
collagen vascular disease	5 (8%)	8 (12%)
HIV infection	4 (6%)	5 (8%)
NYHA classification		
II	48%	51%
III	52%	49%
Six-min walk test mean (m)	362 ± 94	383 ± 93
Hemodynamic parameters		
right atrial pressure (mmHg)	7.9 ± 5.4	8.6 ± 5.5
mean PAP (mmHg)	57.8 ± 21.2	$60.6 + 15.3$
cardiac index (l/min/m^2)	2.4 ± 0.7	2.4 ± 0.7
PVR index (units/m^2)	22.7 ± 12.8	23.9 ± 10.8

PPH, primary pulmonary hypertension; PAP, pulmonary arterial pressure; PVR, pulmonary venous resistance

Patients were randomized to placebo or beraprost sodium (20 μg tablets) and the daily dose was titrated weekly over a 6-week period to a maximum tolerated dose of 80–480 μg per day, delivered as four equal split doses. From weeks 7 to 12, the maximum tolerated dose was maintained.

Changes in the primary endpoint in this study, which was the 6-min walk test, showed an improvement of 15 m in the active treatment group, compared with a decline of 10 m in the placebo group, giving an overall treatment effect of 25 m, which is statistically significant ($p = 0.036$; see Table 8). Some baseline characteristics interacted with the treatment effect in the 6-min walk test, but there was no effect of NYHA functional class, showing that beraprost sodium is equally effective in classes II and III. In contrast, etiology was shown to have an important effect, with beraprost being much more effective for PPH than non-PPH, for which there was no statistically significant effect (Figure 3). It is notable that there was no deterioration in clinical state after 12 weeks in the APH placebo group, suggesting that these patients were more stable than those with PPH.

There was a significant and clinically important improvement in the Borg dyspnea index in the treatment group, compared with a deterioration in the placebo group (Figure 4). There was also a trend to an improvement in NYHA functional class and cardiopulmonary hemodynamic variables under beraprost sodium. As expected, in a trial that included many patients in the early stages of PAH, there were few severe critical events, with only one death in each group and a few admissions to hospital (Table 9). Most of the treatment-related adverse events were related to the study drug, as observed with other prostacyclin

TABLE 8   Changes from baseline to week 12 in the 6-min walk test. Where appropriate, data are given as mean ± standard deviation

	Beraprost sodium ($n = 65$)	Placebo ($n = 65$)
Distance at baseline (m)	362 ± 94	383 ± 93
Distance at week 12 (m)	377 ± 113	374 ± 121
Change from baseline (m)	15 ± 8	−10 ± 8
Treatment effect		
mean	+25 m	
95% CI	1.8–48.32	
p value	0.036	

Missing data imputation by last observation carried forward

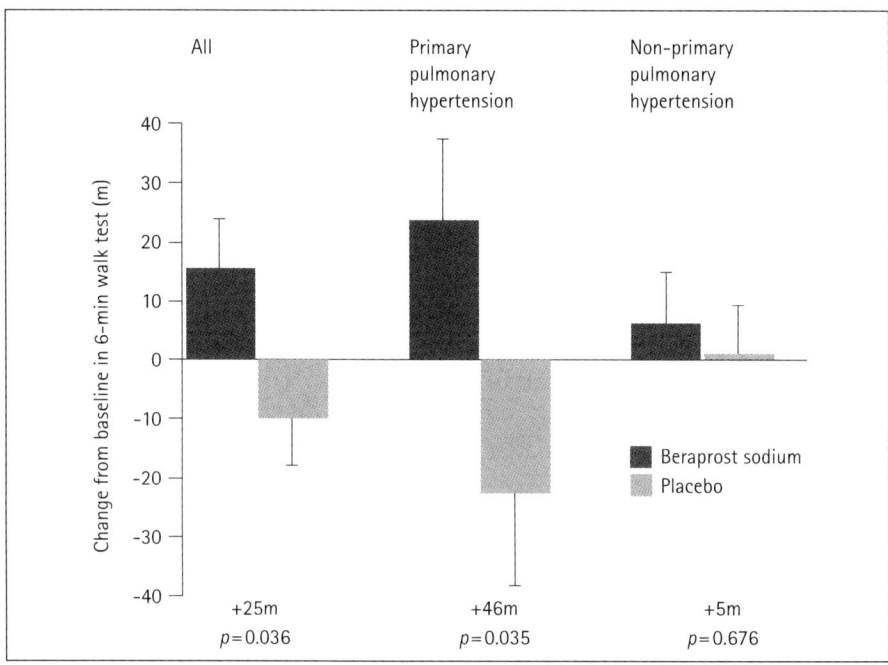

FIGURE 3   Treatment effect of beraprost sodium and placebo on exercise capacity at week 12 in all subjects and subgroups with primary and non-primary pulmonary hypertension[8]

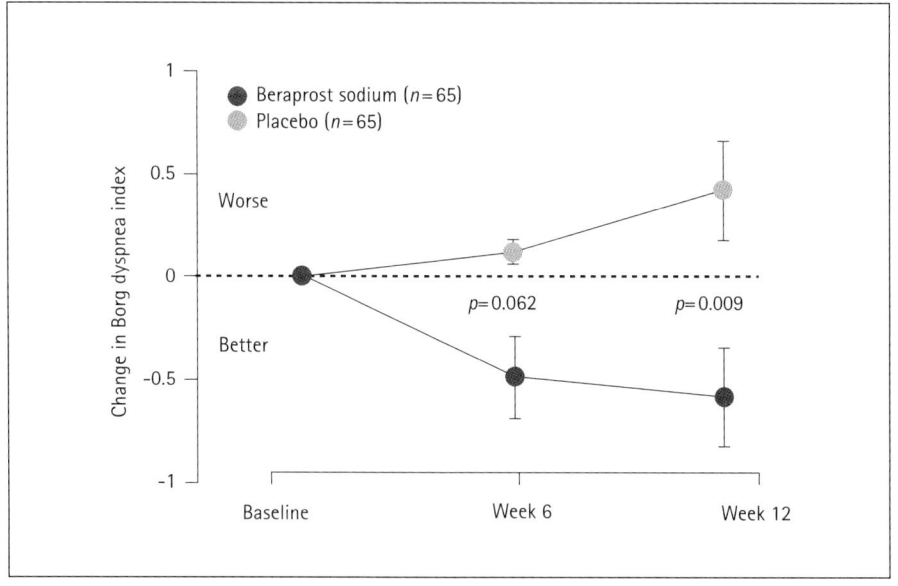

FIGURE 4   Borg dyspnea index at baseline and weeks 6 and 12 in treatment and placebo groups, showing a beneficial effect of beraprost sodium[8]

analogs, but it is noteworthy that the effects were particularly marked during the 6-week titration period, when the maximum tolerated dose was being determined. During the maintenance period (weeks 7–12), the incidence of side-effects was, however, much lower (Table 10). Premature discontinuation of treatment was only required in three patients.

In summary, the ALPHABET trial showed that, in patients with PAH, treatment with beraprost sodium significantly increased exercise capacity and symptoms, compared with placebo. Similar improvements were observed in both NYHA functional classes II and III, and particularly in patients with PPH, in whom a mean improvement in the 6-min walk test of 46 m was observed, which is similar to that seen with intravenous prostacyclin treatment. The safety profile of the drug was excellent, with neither systemic hypotension nor hepatic or renal side-effects. Adverse events were typical of those observed with all prostacyclin analogs (flushing, headache, jaw pain and diarrhea) and were frequent during the dose escalation phase, but were much less frequent during maintenance at the maximum tolerated dose.

TABLE 9   All causes mortality and/or hospitalization for pulmonary arterial hypertension (PAH)

Mortality and hospitalization for deterioration due to PAH	Beraprost sodium ($n = 65$)	Placebo ($n = 65$)	p Value
Mortality	1 (1.5%)	1 (1.5%)	1.00
Combined	4 (6%)	3 (5%)	

TABLE 10   Incidence of treatment-related adverse events according to the study period. Data are presented as percentages

	Beraprost sodium		Placebo	
Events (%)	Titration (weeks 1–6)	Maintenance (weeks 7–12)	Titration (weeks 1–6)	Maintenance (weeks 7–12)
Headache	68	17	17	2
Flushing	54	14	12	5
Jaw pain	28	5	2	0
Diarrhea	26	3	6	2
Leg pain	22	5	6	2
Nausea	20	6	5	3

CONCLUSIONS

The results presented here of the recent large-scale, randomized, placebo-controlled studies of treprostinol and beraprost sodium for the treatment of PAH[7,8] suggest that stable prostacyclin analogs administered subcutaneously or orally are effective and safe, and offer clinicians novel, less invasive alternatives to intravenous prostacyclin for the treatment of this devastating and life-threatening condition.

REFERENCES

1. Rubin LJ. Pathology and pathophysiology of primary pulmonary hypertension. *Am J Cardiol* 1995;75:51–4A

2. Christman BW, McPherson CD, Newman JH, *et al.* An imbalance between the excretion of thromboxane and prostacyclin metabolites in pulmonary hypertension. *N Engl J Med* 1992;327:70–5

3. Barst RJ, Rubin LJ, Long WA, *et al.* A comparison of continuous intravenous epoprostenol (prostacyclin) with conventional therapy for primary pulmonary hypertension. The Primary Pulmonary Hypertension Study Group. *N Engl J Med* 1996;334:296–302

4. Badesch DB, Tapson VF, McGoon MD, *et al.* Continuous intravenous epoprostenol for pulmonary hypertension due to the scleroderma spectrum of disease. A randomized, controlled trial. *Ann Intern Med* 2000;132:425–34

5. Rich S, Kaufmann E, Levy PS. The effect of high doses of calcium-channel blockers on survival in primary pulmonary hypertension. *N Engl J Med* 1992;327:76–81

6. Barst RJ. Treatment of primary pulmonary hypertension with continuous intravenous prostacyclin. *Heart* 1997;77:299–301

7. Simonneau G, Barst RJ, Galiè N, *et al.* Continuous subcutaneous infusion of treprostinil, a prostacyclin analogue, in patients with pulmonary arterial hypertension. *Am J Respir Crit Care Med* 2002;165:800–4

8. Galiè N, Humbert M, Vachiéry J-C, *et al.* Effects of beraprost sodium, an oral prostacyclin analogue, in patients with pulmonary arterial hypertension: a randomized, double-blind, placebo-controlled trial. *J Am Coll Cardiol* 2002;39:1496–502

DISCUSSION

Professor Higenbottam (Sheffield, UK)

I note that, with the oral prostanoid, there is apparently benefit in the earlier stages of the disease, in terms of the NYHA functional class, and I wonder what the mechanisms are and why this should be different from systemic therapy?

Professor Simonneau

I think systemic administration is not a problem if there are no side-effects from the drug. I'm sure that the ideal treatment for patients is oral therapy and, although subcutaneous injection and inhalation are not invasive, or only minimally invasive, they are not very convenient for the patient. We need to develop our treatment because, at the early stage of the disease, the patient can accept more non-invasive therapy.

Professor Higenbottam

I just wondered whether the worry about the intravenous infusion lines and the complications of the lines actually contributes in some way to the disease itself. That was my anxiety when we started on our program and one of the reasons we omitted patients with the earlier stages of the disease in selecting patients for treatment. We can't answer that question with regard to the oral therapy, but there is perhaps a hint that a less invasive route does not contribute so much to progression.

Professor Simonneau

But actually the patient at the early stage of the disease needs some effective therapy because, even in NYHA class I or II, the majority of patients will progress within a few years. It's very important to prevent this deterioration of the disease.

Unknown questioner

Given the data presented on the efficacy of intravenous prostacyclin, I wondered why that wasn't used as one of the comparison groups in the studies?

Professor Simonneau

It was impossible to carry out these trials in a double-blind fashion with intravenous prostacyclin.

Non–prostacyclin therapeutic options for treating pulmonary hypertension

N. Galiè, A. Manes, M. Aquilina and A. Branzi

We have waited for many decades for new treatments for pulmonary arterial hypertension (PAH). Until recently, the only treatment for PAH was symptomatic and based on empiric experience and/or uncontrolled trials[1]. 'Conventional' treatment included oral anticoagulants, calcium channel blockers (in the minority of patients who respond to acute pharmacologic challenge, i.e. 15–25% of cases, depending on the definition of response), diuretics, digoxin and oxygen. In the 1990s, three randomized studies[2–4] provided a rational basis for treating PAH, by demonstrating that the continuous intravenous infusion of prostacyclin, a vasodilator and antiproliferative agent, improved functional capacity, cardiopulmonary hemodynamics and survival in patients in NYHA functional classes III and IV with primary pulmonary hypertension (PPH) or PAH associated with scleroderma. Since then, intravenous prostacyclin has become the reference treatment for advanced PAH, either as a bridge to transplantation, or as an alternative treatment. However, the treatment requires permanent intravenous catheters and portable infusion pumps; it is associated with potentially life-threatening complications and a range of troublesome side-effects. For all these reasons, effective alternatives to intravenous prostacyclin for PAH have been sought, including analogs which can be administered subcutaneously (treprostinol) or orally (beraprost sodium), as discussed in detailed in Chapter 3, or by inhalation, as described for iloprost in Chapters 5 and 6.

METABOLIC ABNORMALITIES IN PAH

The rationale for the administration of prostacyclin, a vasodilator produced by vascular endothelial cells, is that, in PAH, the metabolic pathways leading to prostacyclin are dysregulated (Figure 1). Indeed, it has been shown that patients with PAH excrete lower levels of urinary metabolites of prostacyclin and their arteries have a lower expression of prostacyclin synthase[5]. In addition, thromboxane levels are increased in these patients. Overall, the biochemical pathophysiology of PAH is, however, more complex and involves the dysregulation of three main pathways, namely, the prostacyclin pathway itself, the nitric oxide pathway, and the endothelin pathway. Some studies also show a reduction in nitric oxide synthase in PAH, whilst others show an increase, so we do not know if the availability of nitric oxide in this disease is reduced or unchanged. It is known that endothelin-1 is increased in PAH, leading to vasoconstriction and proliferation. All these systems are dysregulated in patients with the disease and provide a wide range of alternative approaches to treatment.

The thromboxane synthase inhibitor and receptor antagonist, terbogrel, was the subject of the first randomized study of oral treatment of PPH. Exogenous prostacyclin can, of course, be given by various routes. Inhaled nitric oxide can also be used for treatment, and the NO precursor L-arginine may also be effective. Cyclic guanosine monophosphate (cGMP), which mediates the activity of nitric oxide, is degraded by phosphodiesterase-5 (PDE-5),

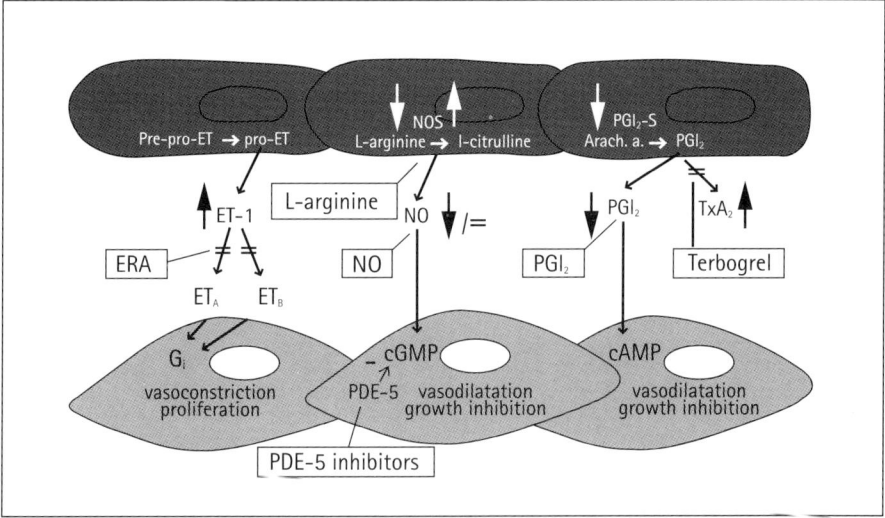

FIGURE 1   Endothelial dysfunction in PAH and strategies for correction, as indicated by white boxes. See text for further details

which is itself inhibited by certain compounds, leading to enhancement of nitric oxide activity. In addition, endothelin-1 receptor antagonists (ERAs) can be used. All these alternatives for the treatment of PAH will now be reviewed.

THROMBOXANE INHIBITION WITH PROSTACYCLIN STIMULATION

PPH is known to exhibit an imbalance in the production of thromboxane and prostacyclin, which have the same precursor, arachidonic acid, so that thromboxane is produced at the expense of prostacyclin. The first attempts at non-prostacyclin therapy of PPH were with the combined thromboxane synthetase inhibitor/receptor antagonist terbogrel[6]. Unfortunately, the trial had to be stopped because there was an unacceptable incidence of the unexpected side-effect of leg pain. This was not harmful by itself but impaired determination of the primary endpoint of the trial, namely, exercise capacity. However, the pathophysiological rationale of the study was vindicated, because terbogrel was shown to reduce circulating thromboxane and to increase endogenous prostacyclin production.

ENDOTHELIN-1 RECEPTOR ANTAGONISTS

Endothelin-1 is produced by vascular endothelial cells and is the most potent endogenous vasoconstrictor yet discovered[7]. By acting on the promoter gene for endothelin-1, various agents and other factors stimulate its production, including pulsatile stress, shear stress, pH, hypoxia, angiotensin II, thrombin, cytokines and growth factors. Two distinct endothelin-1 receptors, ET_A and ET_B, have been identified on almost all types of cell, including vascular smooth muscle cells, where they mediate contraction and proliferation. Endothelin-1 plasma levels are increased in almost all forms of pulmonary hypertension (Table 1) and are closely related to hemodynamic changes (Figure 2)[8] and prognosis (Figure 3)[9].

Early attempts to modify endothelin-1 levels used endothelin-converting enzyme inhibitors (ECE-I), the rationale being similar to that of angiotensin-converting enzyme inhibitors (ACE-I). However, an ECE-I was found to be ineffective because the production of endothelin-1 depends on several isoforms of the enzymes (Figure 4). Hence, endothelin-1 receptor antagonists (ERAs) that block both endothelin-1 receptors were developed, using both peptide and non-peptide drugs[10]. ERAs prevent and even reverse pathologic and hemodynamic changes in experimental models of both hypoxia and monocrotaline-induced PAH. These favorable laboratory results recently prompted clinical trials involving patients with primary PH or PH associated with scleroderma. Treatment with the oral ERA bosentan

TABLE 1   Endothelin-1 plasma levels are increased in conditions with pulmonary hypertension

Primary pulmonary hypertension, persistent pulmonary hypertension of the newborn

CREST (calcinosis, Raynoud's phenomenon, esophageal dysfunction, sclerodactyly, telangiectasia)

Eisenmenger syndrome

Mitral stenosis

Congestive heart failure

Chronic obstructive pulmonary disease, interstitial pulmonary fibrosis

High-altitude exposure

Obstructive sleep apnea

Pulmonary hypertension after heart surgery

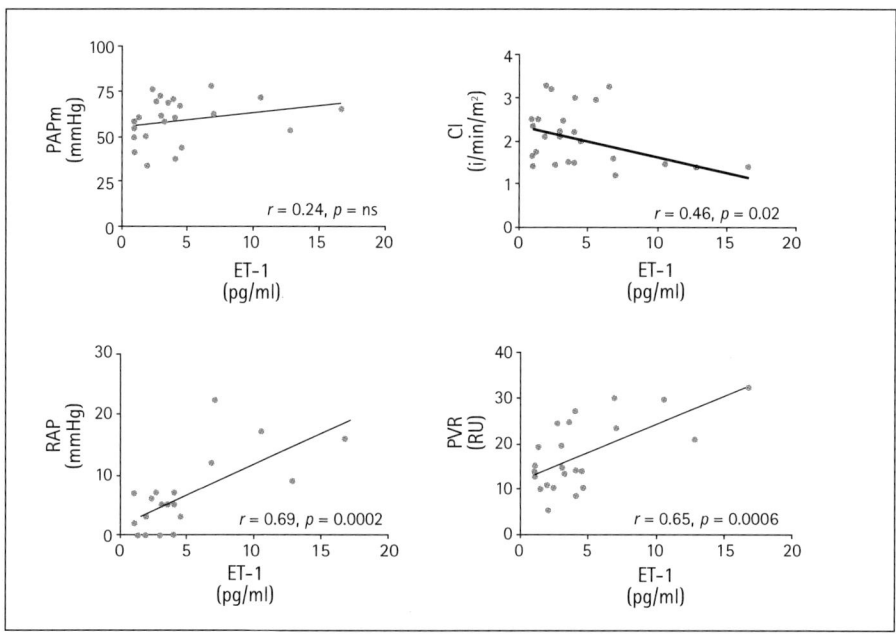

FIGURE 2   Correlations between levels of endothelin-1 and hemodynamic variables in PPH[8]

has been shown to be effective in terms of symptoms, exercise capacity, clinical events and cardiopulmonary hemodynamics.

In a recent 12-week pilot study, a group of 32 patients with PPH were randomized to bosentan (125 mg twice a day) or placebo. Active treatment showed a marked improvement in

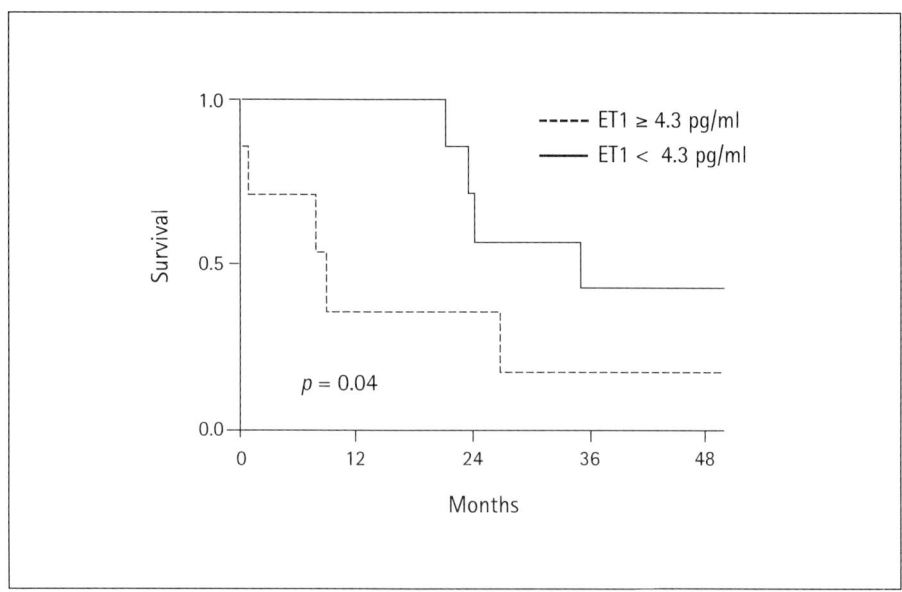

FIGURE 3   Log rank comparison of survival of patients with PPH according to endothelin-1 levels[9]

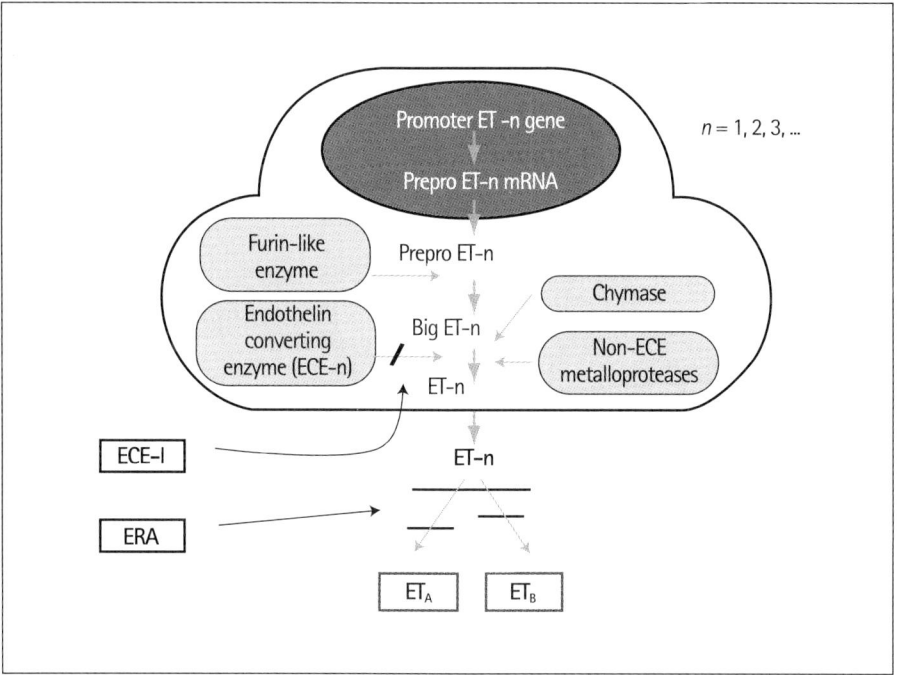

FIGURE 4   Endothelin-1 pathways and strategies for blocking them, indicated by a bar across the pathway. See the text for further details

exercise capacity according to the 6-min walk test, and reductions in mean PAP and cardiac index[11] (Figure 5). These encouraging results led to the BREATHE-1 study, which was carried out with 217 patients randomized to placebo or one of two doses of bosentan, namely, 125 mg or 250 mg twice daily[12]. In the groups treated with these different doses of bosentan, there was an improvement in the 6-min walk test, compared with a progressive deterioration in the placebo group. After 16 weeks' treatment with bosentan, exercise capacity was increased by 45 meters. Moreover, the clinical deterioration of the bosentan-treated population was slower than that of the placebo group. Bosentan was also associated with remodelling of the heart, increasing the size of the left ventricle and decreasing that of the right ventricle[13]. These observations are of considerable interest, as they were seen after only 16 weeks of treatment, and it seems likely that chronic bosentan treatment may achieve even further remodelling of the heart chambers.

ENHANCING NITRIC OXIDE LEVELS

Nitric oxide (NO) is a simple molecule which acts as an important regulator of vascular tone and is produced by endothelial cells. It is generated by the conversion of L-arginine to

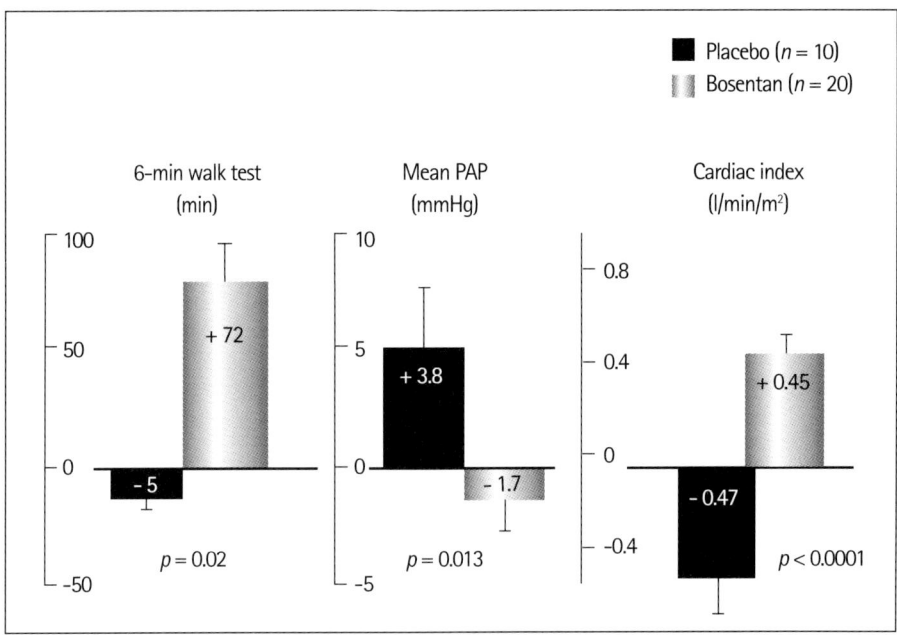

FIGURE 5   Changes in exercise capacity, mean PAP and cardiac index in patients with PPH treated with the ERA bosentan or placebo[11]

L-citrulline under the influence of nitric oxide synthase (Figure 1), a process that is stimulated physiologically by the biochemical mediators thrombin, adenosine diphosphate, and bradykinin, and physicochemically by the stimuli of shear stress. Once produced, NO diffuses from endothelial cells to smooth muscle cells, which it induces to relax by activating guanylate cyclase, which in turn promotes the production of cyclic guanosine monophosphate (cGMP). NO also inhibits the growth of smooth muscle cells.

The classic study of Pepka-Zaba and colleagues[14] demonstrated the exquisite pulmonary selectivity of NO by showing that it reduced pulmonary vascular resistance without altering systemic vascular resistance (Figure 6). The involvement of NO in PAH has been demonstrated in the endothelial cells of patients, which have been shown to contain lower than normal levels of nitric oxide synthase, suggesting that the vascular abnormalities of the disease could be due, at least partially, to insufficient NO[15]. In support of this, the acute administration of NO to PAH patients[16] reduced pulmonary arterial pressure (PAP), whilst

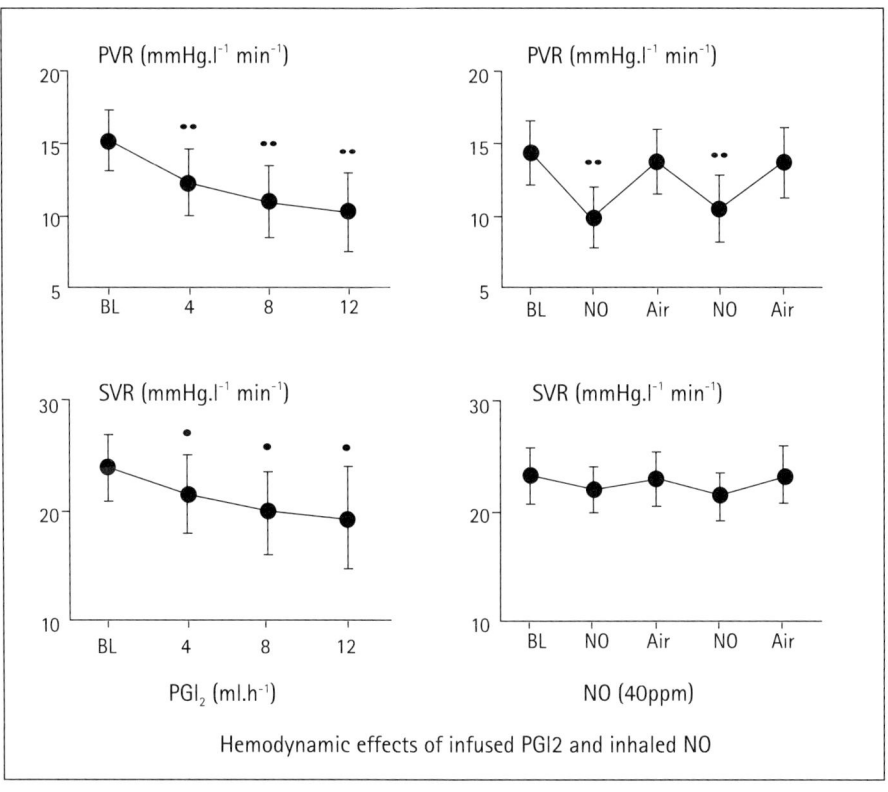

FIGURE 6   Effects of infused prostacyclin and inhaled NO on PVR and SVR in patients with PPH[14]

chronic administration has been reported to give favorable results, albeit in a small series[17] (Table 2). Newly developed portable NO sources using nasal prongs may offer a solution to the practical problems of chronic administration, but this promising approach needs further evaluation in a controlled clinical trial.

NO production rates can also be increased by administering supplements of the nitric oxide synthase substrate L-arginine (Figure 7). In animal models of PH, such supplements have been shown to increase endothelium-derived vasodilation, whilst, in neonates, a deficiency of L-arginine and L-citrulline, and low levels of urinary NO metabolites are known to be associated with persistent PAH[18] (Figure 8). A recent placebo-controlled study showed that acute supplementation with L-arginine in PPH patients can, indeed, reduce mean PAP and

TABLE 2 Hemodynamic data at baseline and after 15 min of inhalation of NO via the pulsed delivery device*

Patient	PAPm (mmHg)	RAPm (mmHg)	CO (l/min)	PCWP (mmHg)	PVR (dyne.s.cm^{-5})	MAP (mmHg)	SVR (dyne.s.cm^{-5})
1. Baseline	51	7	5.7	10	577	100	1305
NO	47	2	5.7	10	522	91	1247
2. Baseline	33	1	3.8	5	579	88	1798
NO	29	1	4.4	6	415	95	1715
3. Baseline	41	5	6.7	9	378	87	968
NO	35	5	7.5	9	277	80	800
4. Baseline	49	4	3.7	10	850	95	1984
NO	45	3	3.4	10	821	93	2111
5. Baseline	45	21	2.1	9	1385	111	3461
NO	33	17	2.2	9	881	100	3046
6. Baseline	75	16	5.7	7	949	102	1218
NO	59	14	6.2	8	658	95	1045
7. Baseline	56	13	5.3	8	728	92	1199
NO	44	8	6.0	8	483	70	1181
8. Baseline	60	10	4.9	10	821	87	1265
NO	53	9	5.2	7	708	97	1354
Mean ± SD							
Baseline	51 ± 12	9 ± 6.6	4.7 ± 1.4	8.5 ± 1.8	790 ± 285	95 ± 8	1688 ± 763
NO	43 ± 10*	6.6 ± 5.6**	4.9 ± 1.7	8.3 ± 1.3	620 ± 208**	90 ± 10	1624 ± 701

RAPm = mean right atrial pressure; MAP = mean arterial pressure; PCWP = pulmonary capillary wedge pressure

*$p = 0.001$ NO vs. baseline; **$p = 0.01$ NO vs. baseline

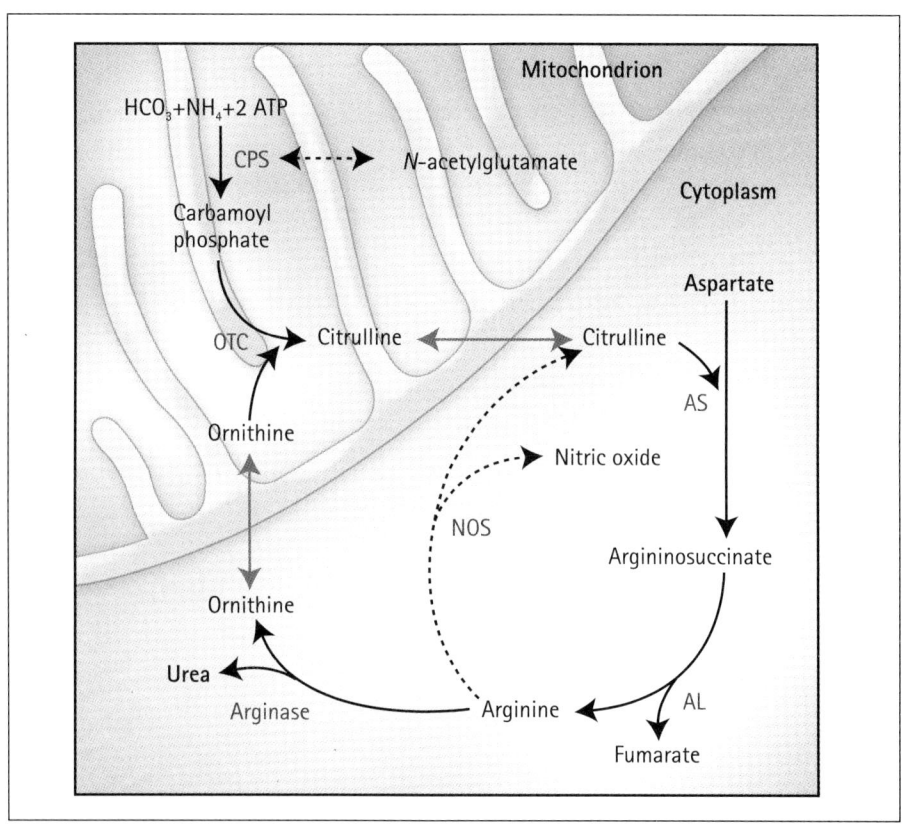

FIGURE 7   Metabolic pathways involving NO[18]

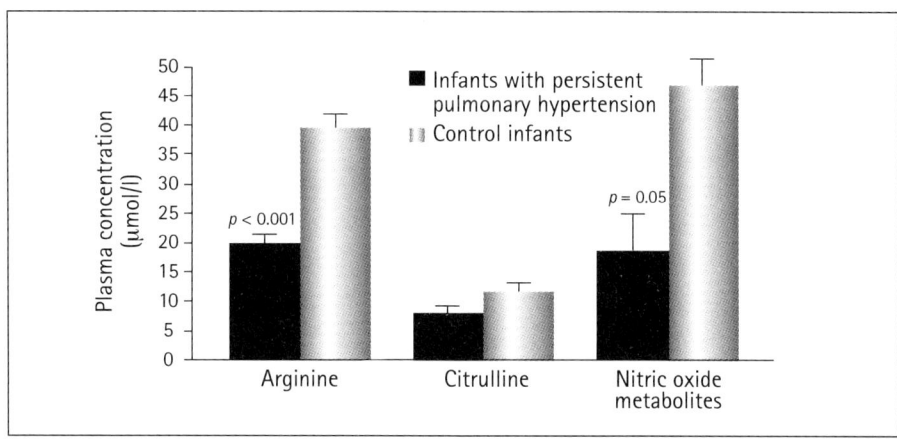

FIGURE 8   Comparison of plasma concentrations of L-arginine, L-citrulline, and NO metabolites in infants with persistent PH and controls[18]

increase the cardiac index, leading to a reduction in calculated PVR (Figures 9 and 10)[19]. After only 1 week of treatment, there was an increase in peak VO_2, compared with a small reduction in the placebo group. Although the results of L-arginine supplementation are, therefore, promising, a large-scale clinical trial is required to confirm the preliminary findings.

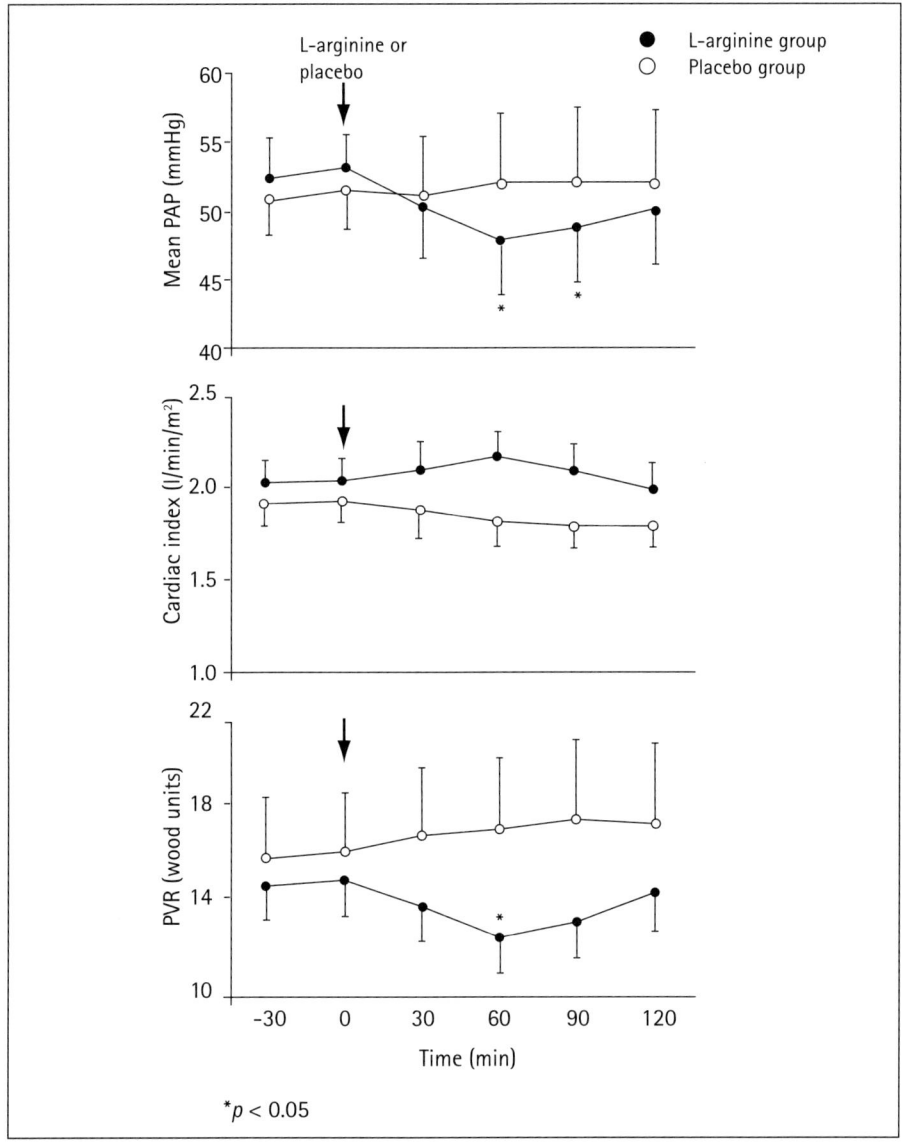

FIGURE 9   Effects of acute L-arginine supplementation on mean PAP, PVR and cardiac index in patients with PPH[19]

Sildenafil is an orally active, potent, selective inhibitor of cGMP-specific phosphodiesterase type 5, which is the predominant phosphodiesterase isoenzyme in human corpora cavernosa and is particularly abundant in the pulmonary vasculature, but not in systemic vessels (Figure 11). Sildenafil, which is probably best known as the active ingredient of the anti-impotence drug Viagra®, increases the concentration of NO-derived cGMP, thereby enhancing the effects of NO; it would be expected to reverse the metabolic and vascular defects of low levels of NO in PAH patients. Similar results to those obtained with supplementation with NO or L-arginine can be obtained with PDE-5 inhibitors, which inhibit the degradation of cGMP by PDE-5. Preliminary results with sildenafil, given intravenously to PPH

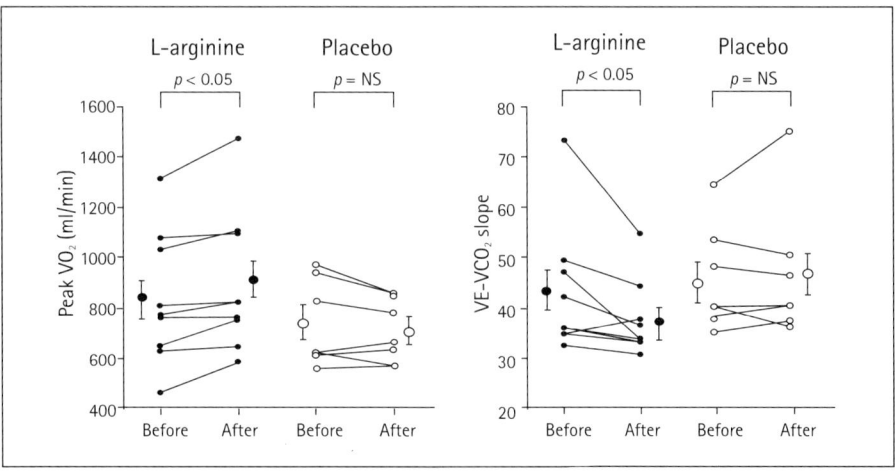

FIGURE 10 Effects of 1 week of L-arginine supplementation on respiratory variables in patients with PPH[19]. Large circles represent mean values

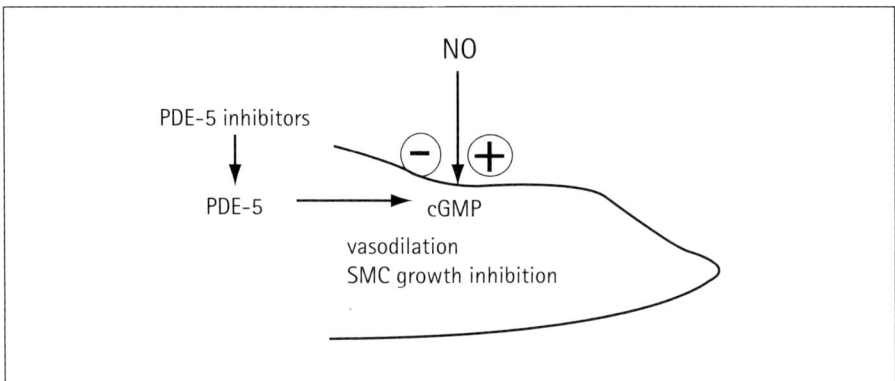

FIGURE 11 Schematic diagram showing the mode of action of PDE-5 inhibitors

patients at increasing doses, show a progressive decrease in PVR, similar to that obtained by inhalation of NO (unpublished data). Preliminary results, presented by T.E. Siddons at the American Thoracic Society Meeting in 2001, show that the chronic administration of sildenafil in PAH patients for a period of 3 months increases exercise capacity and reduces PVR (Figure 12). Other favorable reports in pediatric PPH are also available[20]. A randomized clinical study is now required to determine the effects of this drug in a larger group of patients.

NON–MEDICAL TREATMENT

Despite the promise of medical approaches to PAH, it should always be remembered that there are alternative non-pharmacologic interventional approaches to treatment, which are indicated when patients fail to respond to medical treatment. These include graded balloon atrial septostomy (GBAT), which seems to increase survival[21] (Figure 13), and lung transplantation, which is a treatment of last resort and may be effective with advanced disease. GBAT is an invasive procedure that is intended to create an intra-atrial defect, in order to effect a right-to-left shunt of blood flow. Experimental and clinical observations suggest that, as expected, such an intervention can reduce right atrial pressure and increase systemic output, thereby improving exercise capacity and survival[21]. GBAT is performed by means of the transeptal technique of Brockenbrough, with the stepwise use of multiple balloons of increasing size, employed to achieve a dilatation that produces a fall in systemic oxygen

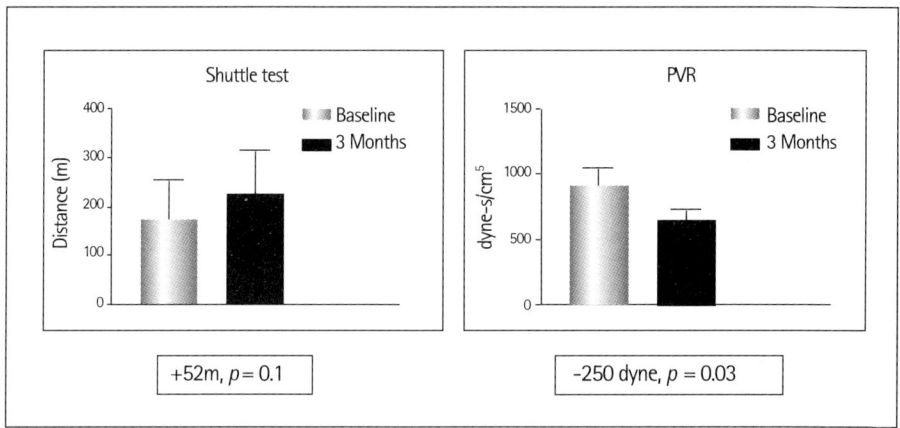

FIGURE 12   Effect of 3 months' therapy with sildenafil (25 mg three times a day) on PVR and exercise capacity in four patients with PAH. Adapted from Siddons TE, 2001 Meeting of the American Thoracic Society

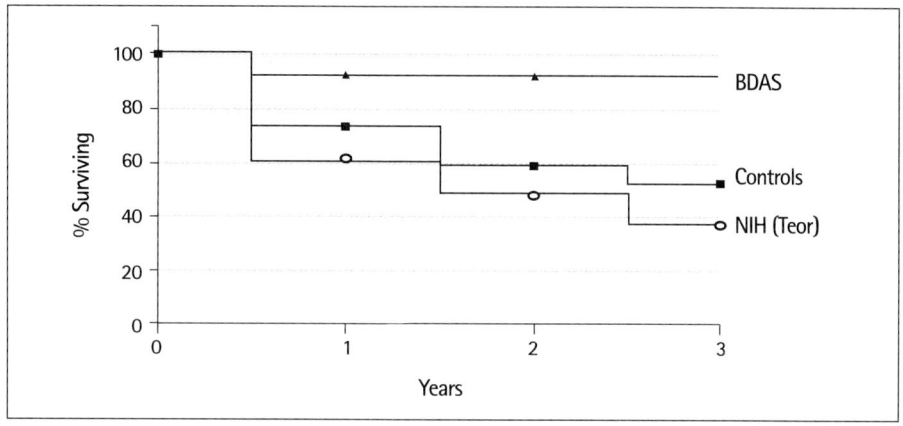

FIGURE 13 Survival after graded balloon dilation atrial septostomy in patients with severe pulmonary hypertension, compared with controls and with expected survival based on NIH Registry prognostic formula[21]

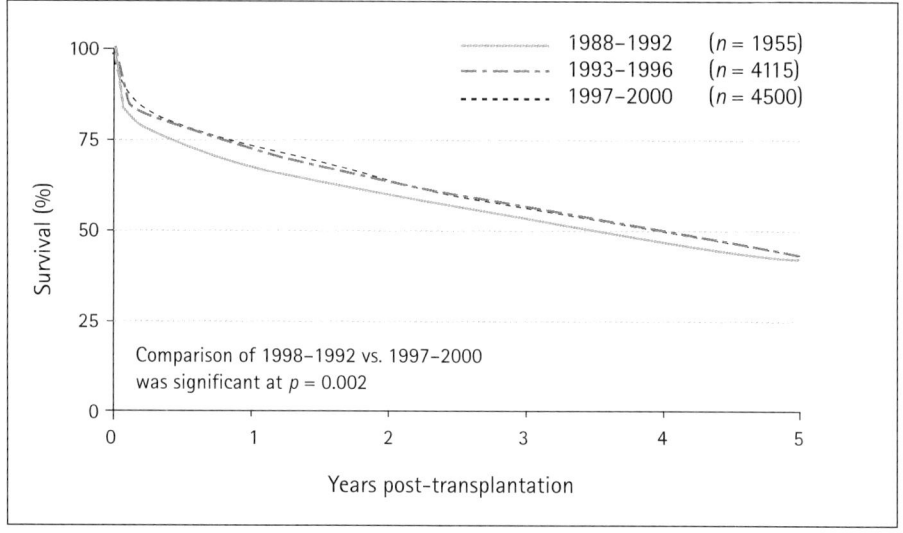

FIGURE 14 Actuarial survival (1988–2000) after adult lung transplantation[22]

saturation of not more than 5–10%. Procedure-related failure and death are not negligible, however, and GBAT should only be performed in centers with experience in both interventional cardiology and PAH.

The results of heart and heart–lung transplantation have improved in recent years, so that the global survival after lung transplantation for all indications now rests at approximately

70%, 62% and 55% after 1, 2 and 3 years, respectively[22] (Figure 14). Conversely, a diagnosis of PAH increases the risks of death within 1 year, whilst long waiting lists further reduce potential benefits. For these reasons, the transplantation of both lungs and heart is indicated where medical therapy fails.

CONCLUSIONS

The availability of many alternative therapeutic options for PAH should, in the near future, allow the optimal strategy to be tailored for each patient. The 'best drug' for treating PAH probably does not exist and the most appropriate drug, or perhaps combination of drugs, needs to be determined for each patient. This is the real challenge for the future in the treatment of all forms of pulmonary hypertension.

REFERENCES

1.   Galiè N. Do we need controlled clinical trials in pulmonary arterial hypertension? *Eur Respir J* 2001;17:1–3

2.   Rubin LJ, Mendoza J, Hood M, *et al*. Treatment of primary pulmonary hypertension with continuous intravenous prostacyclin (epoprostenol). Results of a randomized trial. *Ann Intern Med* 1990;112:485–91

3.   Barst RJ, Rubin LJ, McGoon MD, Caldwell EJ, Long WA, Levy PS. Survival in primary pulmonary hypertension with long-term continuous intravenous prostacyclin. *Ann Intern Med* 1994;121:409–15

4.   Barst RJ, Rubin LJ, Long WA, *et al*. A comparison of continuous intravenous epoprostenol (prostacyclin) with conventional therapy for primary pulmonary hypertension. The Primary Pulmonary Hypertension Study Group. *N Engl J Med* 1996;334:296–302

5.   Tuder RM, Cool CD, Geraci MW, *et al*. Prostacyclin synthase expression is decreased in lungs from patients with severe pulmonary hypertension. *Am J Respir Crit Care Med* 1999;159:1925–32

6.   Langleben D, Christman BW, Barst RJ, *et al*. Effects of the thromboxane synthetase inhibitor and receptor antagonist, terbogrel, in patients with primary pulmonary hypertension. *Am Heart J* 2002; in press

7.   Yanagisawa M. The endothelin system. A new target for therapeutic intervention. *Circulation* 1994;89:1320–2

8. Galiè N, Borgatti ML, Ussia GP, *et al*. Comparative relation of neurohormonal activation to hemodynamics in primary or precapillary secondary pulmonary hypertension. *J Am Coll Cardiol* 1995;25:40A

9. Galie N, Grigioni F, Bacchi-Reggiani L, *et al*. Relation of endothelin-1 to survival in patients with primary pulmonary hypertension. *Eur J Clin Invest* 1996;26:141

10. Luscher TF, Barton M. Endothelins and endothelin receptor antagonists: therapeutic considerations for a novel class of cardiovascular drugs. *Circulation* 2000;102:2434–40

11. Channick RN, Simonneau G, Sitbon O, *et al*. Effects of the dual endothelin-receptor antagonist bosentan in patients with pulmonary hypertension: a randomised placebo-controlled study. *Lancet* 2001;358:1119–23

12. Rubin LJ, Badesch DB, Barst R, *et al*. Bosentan therapy in patients with pulmonary arterial hypertension. *N Engl J Med* 2002; in press

13. Galiè N, Hinderliter A, Torbicki A, *et al*. Effects of the oral endothelin receptor antagonist bosentan on echocardiographic and doppler measures in patients with pulmonary arterial hypertension. *J Am Coll Cardiol* 2002; in press.

14. Pepka-Zaba J, Higenbottam TW, Dinh-Xuan AT, Stone D, Wallwork J. Inhaled nitric oxide as a cause of selective pulmonary vasodilatation in pulmonary hypertension. *Lancet* 1991;38:1173–4

15. Giaid A. Nitric oxide and endothelin-1 in pulmonary hypertension. *Chest* 1998;114:208–12S

16. Hoeper MM, Olschewski H, Ghofrani HA, *et al*. A comparison of the acute hemodynamic effects of inhaled nitric oxide and aerosolized iloprost in primary pulmonary hypertension. *J Am Coll Cardiol* 2000;35:176–82

17. Channick RN, Newhart JW, Johnson FW, *et al*. Pulsed delivery of inhaled nitric oxide to patients with primary pulmonary hypertension: an ambulatory delivery system and initial clinical tests. *Chest* 1996;109:1545–9

18. DL Pearson, Dawling S, Walsh WF, *et al*. Neonatal typertension – urea-cycle intermediates, nitric oxide production, and carbamoyl-phosphate synthetase function. *N Engl J Med* 2001;344:1832–8

19. Nagaya N, Uematsu M, Oya H, *et al*. Short-term oral administration of L-arginine improves hemodynamics and exercise capacity in patients with precapillary pulmonary hypertension. *Am J Respir Crit Care Med* 2001;163:887–91

20. Prasad S, Wilkinson J, Gatzoulis MA. Sildenafil in primary pulmonary hypertension. *N Engl J Med* 2000;343:1342

21.   Sandoval J, Gaspar J, Pulido T, *et al.* Graded balloon dilation atrial septostomy in severe primary pulmonary hypertension. A therapeutic alternative for patients nonresponsive to vasodilator treatment. *J Am Coll Cardiol* 1998;32:297–304

22.   UNOS/ISMLT International Regulations for Thoracic Organ Transplant, 2001

DISCUSSION

Professor Higenbottam

A speaker asked a question about the comparison between prostanoids and some of these other therapies. I'd just like to pose the question again to Professor Galiè, because I think the comparison with another treatment is quite an important issue. I recognize the need for placebo-controlled randomized trials, but I guess we're now looking to do comparative studies and I'd be very interested on your thoughts on that.

Professor Galiè

I think that when we had only prostacyclin treatment there was a precise exclusion criterion in trials. The patients who needed prostacyclin were excluded. In fact, the indication for intravenous prostacyclin was NYHA advanced class III and class IV and, in all these trials, the patients obviously, for ethical reasons, were excluded. But now other treatments have shown efficacy. So do we need now to compare the additional new treatments with placebo or with those treatments yet proved effective? It's a very difficult question, because all these treatments are not available to the great majority of practitioners, since they have not yet been approved. Possibly in a year's time, all these treatments will be available, but not now. May be there is a time window within which we can perform placebo-controlled studies, before the drugs are freely available, after which it will be ethically difficult to perform such studies.

5

Physiological benefits of inhaled prostanoids

W. Seeger

INTRODUCTION

Inhaled therapy for pulmonary hypertension (PH) is a fascinating concept that may provide selective targeting of the lung vasculature, thereby avoiding systemic side-effects. This chapter presents the background to this approach, which has been used in a recent controlled, randomized trial of inhaled iloprost (the AIR study), which is reported in Chapter 6.

Selective pulmonary vasodilation has been described for inhaled nitric oxide (NO), but this agent has several disadvantages. Most importantly, there are no data that demonstrate improved survival with inhaled NO. In contrast, there is very strong evidence that prostacyclin (epoprostenol) has a beneficial role in severe primary pulmonary hypertension (PPH), improving survival, exercise capacity, and cardiopulmonary hemodynamics[1-3]. Continuous intravenous infusion of prostacyclin for the treatment of PPH has therefore been approved for clinical use in the USA and several European countries. However, the prostacyclin analog, iloprost, is more suited to inhalation than the native compound, because it has a longer plasma half-life. This compound, which was the first prostacyclin analog to be synthesized, is very stable in saline and is effective in low doses. It shares virtually all of the features of prostacyclin, and may have potent antiplatelet properties.

Pulmonary vasoconstriction may be a predominant feature of PPH and, in the minority of patients who have a marked acute pulmonary response to vasodilators, long-term therapy with high-dose calcium channel blockers (CCBs) may be very successful[4]. The remaining patients, however, do not benefit from such therapy and may even develop right ventricular decompensation with CCBs. It is now possible to identify those few patients suitable for high-dose CCBs by testing with inhaled NO[5]. Long-term inhaled NO by itself has also been suggested for treating PPH[6], but the risks of rebound pulmonary hypertension on cessation of therapy, together with toxicity and the possibility of effective treatment of suitable patients with CCBs, limit the clinical role open to inhaled NO therapy. Current clinical experience shows that the vast majority of severely ill patients require prostanoid therapy. If this is unsuccessful, they can be offered atrial septostomy and/or lung transplantation as options of last resort.

BENEFITS AND DISADVANTAGES OF PROSTANOID THERAPY

Prostacyclin is effective for PPH not only because of its vasodilatory functions, but also because of interference with platelet aggregation and impact on leukocytes due to its antiproliferative effects. However, despite the clear-cut benefits of intravenous prostacyclin, it is a relatively expensive therapy and suffers from a significant incidence of practical problems, notably complications associated with the use of a central venous catheter. The dose range used for continuous intravenous infusion of prostacyclin is wide. Although reported success rates differ considerably[7], it undoubtedly has a substantial impact on survival and provides a bridge that allows transplantation to be timed more freely or even cancelled[8]. The results from the longest study published on the use of intravenous prostacyclin showed that the treatment was only successful in improving survival in patients with decompensated right heart failure, whereas patients with a central venous oxygen saturation above 60% did not benefit[9]. This outcome suggests that the only beneficial effect of prostacyclin on mortality is right ventricular decompensation and that the proposed long-term effects on pulmonary vascular remodelling are offset by the life-threatening hazards of long-term intravenous therapy. In particular, sepsis and discontinuation of therapy are relatively frequent, due to problems with intravenous lines and/or systemic side-effects, such as jaw pain, systemic hypotension and, in patients with oxygenation deterioration, ventilation/perfusion mismatch. Also, tachyphylaxis may require increases in the administered dose of prostanoid every 2–4 weeks. Attempts to make prostanoid therapy safer by the use of subcutaneous and oral therapy are considered elsewhere in Chapter 4, but they have undoubtedly been limited by systemic and local side-effects.

THE PRINCIPLES OF INHALATION THERAPY

The pulmonary vasculature is distributed alongside the airways, in a way that places the resistance vessels directly alongside the alveoli (Figure 1). It is clear that the vasodilatory

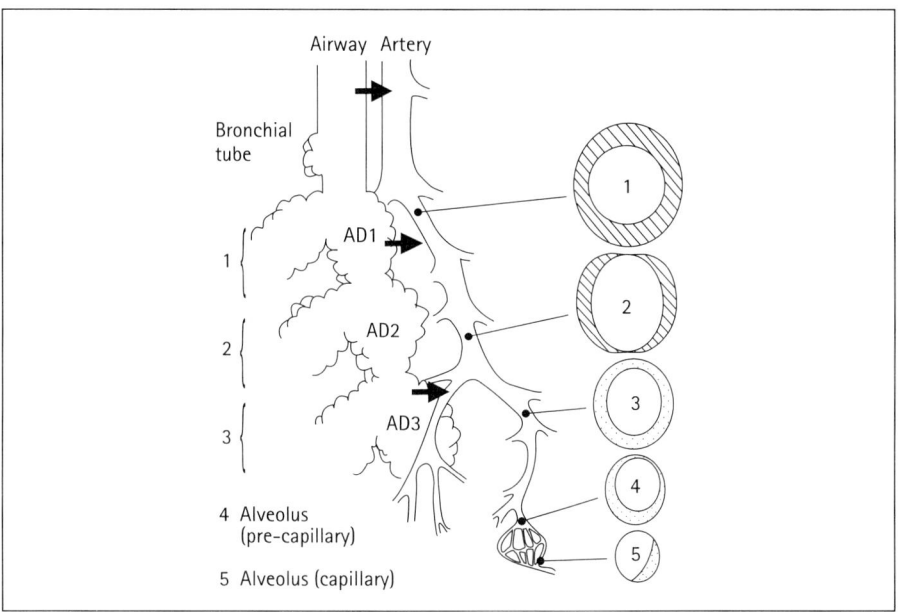

FIGURE 1   The diagram demonstrates the proximity of the pulmonary microvasculature and the small airways[10]

effects of NO are due to the direct effect of this gas on the muscles of the pulmonary vasculature, whereas prostacyclin has both a direct effect on the pulmonary circulation, and a 'spill-over' effect via the general circulation, with recirculation back to the lungs. Some of the disadvantages of intravenous prostanoid therapy might be avoided by the use of a drug which goes directly to the pulmonary circulation. As the intra-acinar pulmonary arteries are closely associated with alveolar surfaces, it is possible to dilate these vessels directly by means of alveolar deposition of drugs. Equally, drugs distributed by inhalation will best affect vessels in close association with ventilated areas and might, therefore, also obviate problems of ventilation/perfusion mismatch. This was the rationale for using inhalation to administer prostacyclin, as first demonstrated for inhaled NO.

PILOT STUDIES OF INHALATION THERAPY

In the early 1990s, interest developed in aerosolizing prostacyclin and delivering it to certain categories of patients, including ventilated patients with respiratory distress syndrome (ARDS), and those with pulmonary hypertension with high shunt flow. Such patients have two major problems with regard to the use of vasodilators (Figure 2). Any drug given

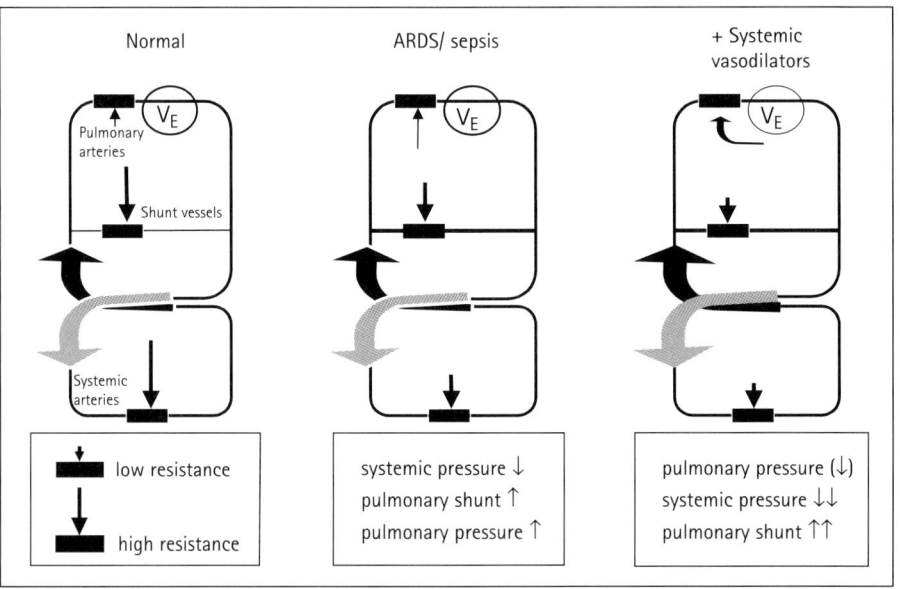

FIGURE 2   Effects of systemic vasodilators in patients with acute respiratory distress syndrome (ARDS)[11]

systemically will achieve vasodilation of the pulmonary vasculature, but at the same time it will vasodilate shunt areas, with the net result of increasing shunt flow. At the same time, systemic vasodilatation is very deleterious for these patients who already have low systemic arterial pressures due to sepsis. In contrast, inhalation of vasodilators achieves a preferential distribution of the drug to the best ventilated areas, thereby avoiding increased shunt flow and a reduction of systemic arterial pressure. In early studies, from 1993 onwards, inhaled prostanoids were shown to achieve a redistribution of blood flow to well-ventilated areas, thereby creating an improvement, rather than a deterioration, in gas exchange[12–14]. Moreover, we found that, in these patients, inhaled prostacyclin had the same pulmonary and intrapulmonary selectivity as inhaled NO.

The first patient treated with inhaled prostacyclin was a severely ill 50-year-old lady with CREST syndrome, with a very high pulmonary artery pressure (PAP) of 75 mmHg, a low cardiac output of 2.5 l/min, and a low central venous oxygen saturation of below 50% (Figure 3a)[15]. After 15 min of inhaled prostacyclin, she responded immediately, with reduction of PAP and an increase in cardiac output, whilst maintaining systemic arterial pressure and without deterioration of gas exchange/arterial oxygenation. The overall effect levelled off within 60–90 min. We then started to use inhaled iloprost, 6 times a day, with good results at 2 years (Figure 3b). Indeed, this first patient is still doing well after 8 years on inhaled iloprost, a stable prostacyclin analog with very similar biological effects to prostacyclin (Figure 4). The plasma half-life of iloprost is 10 times greater than that of prostacyclin, while the therapeutic dose of iloprost is about five-fold lower. Iloprost is chemically

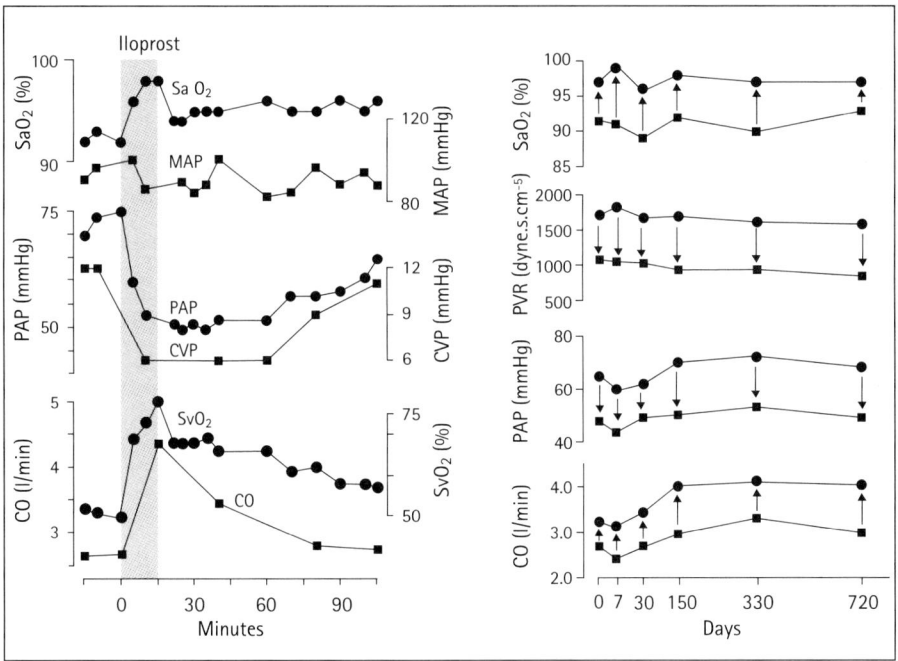

FIGURE 3 Acute and chronic outcomes of inhaled prostacyclin in a 50-year-old female with the CREST syndrome[15]. SaO_2, arterial oxygenation; PAP, pulmonary artery pressure; CO, cardiac output; MAP, mean arterial pressure; CVP, central venous pressure; SvO_2, venous oxygen saturation; PVR, pulmonary vascular resistance

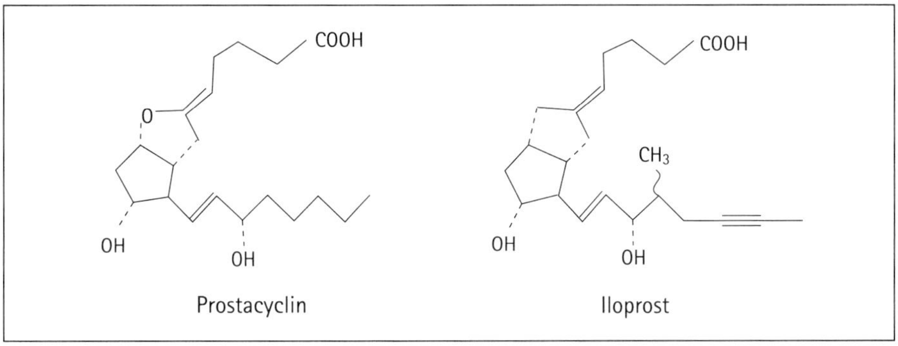

FIGURE 4 Chemical structures of prostacyclin and the stable analog, iloprost

stable in 0.9% NaCL, it has increased antiplatelet properties and possibly a decreased rate of tachyphylaxis.

Following this experience, we carried out a study with six patients with PPH and isolated PH due to collagen vascular disease, comparing intravenous with aerosolized prostacyclin (Table 1)[15]. The pulmonary vascular resistance (PVR) was brought down from 1551 to 1000 dyne.s.cm-5, by titrating the intravenous prostacyclin dose to the maximum tolerable level, and from 1721 to 1019 dyne.s.cm-5, with aerosolized prostacyclin. The decrease in PAP was more prominent with the aerosolized agent and there was also a decrease in the ratio of pulmonary to systemic vascular resistance (SVR), indicating a preferential effect on the pulmonary circulation. Cardiac output improved with both intravenous and aerosolized prostacyclin. Next, we performed further studies comparing inhaled iloprost with inhaled NO and were able to show that aerosolized iloprost is more effective in acutely reducing PVR (Figure 5)[16].

Further developments were, in part, driven by compassionate treatment use. One of the first patients we treated was a 45-year-old woman with severe decompensated heart failure, pleural effusions and shock-like conditions[17]. She had an extremely high PVR, which was higher than the SVR, an extremely low cardiac index of 1.25 l/min/m^2, and a very high PAP

TABLE 1   Acute response to the maximal tolerated dose of intravenous and inhaled PGI2 ($n = 6$)[15]

	Before intravenous PGI2	Intravenous PGI2	Before aerosolized PGI2	Aerosolized PGI2
Pulmonary vascular resistance (dyn.s.cm-5)	1551	1000**	1721	1019**
Pulmonary artery pressure (mmHg)	62.7	59.8	62.3	50.8**
Systemic artery pressure (mmHg)	100	87**	96	90
Pulmonary vascular resistance/ systemic vascular resistance	0.6	0.68	0.67	0.55**
Heart rate (beats/min)	102	107**	102	99
Cardiac output (l/min)	2.94	4.52**	2.75	4.11**

$^* p < 0.05$; $^{**} p < 0.01$

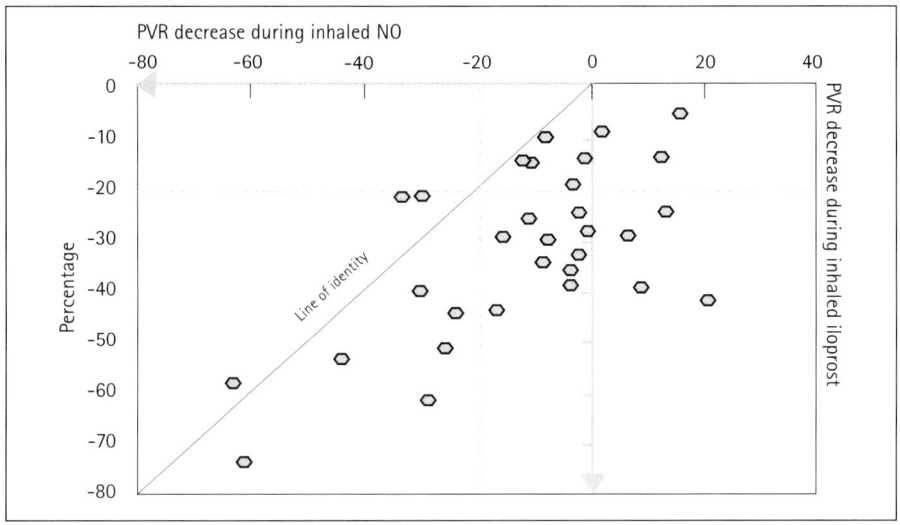

FIGURE 5 Comparison of decrease in pulmonary vascular resistance (PVR) with inhaled NO and inhaled iloprost in severe pulmonary hypertension, showing greater efficacy of prostacyclin[16]

(Table 2a). She responded to some extent to NO. We then tried intravenous prostacyclin, but the treatment was ineffective due to a reduction in arterial pressure, leading to extreme hyperventilation (she was not mechanically ventilated). We then administered inhaled iloprost, which showed a very good acute vasodilatory effect, with a reduction of PVR from 2415 to 1580 dyne.s.cm^{-5} and an increase in cardiac output. She was in a shock-like condition with a low systemic arterial pressure and a negative base excess. The onset of renal failure was evident, with severe liver congestion, an LDH of 2556 U/l and elevated bilirubin (Table 2b). After 1 month of inhaled iloprost therapy, she was able to get up again and, at 6 weeks, her chest radiograph showed signs of improvement. She has now been successfully maintained for several years on inhaled iloprost.

PROSPECTIVE MULTICENTER STUDY OF INHALED ILOPROST FOR DECOMPENSATED RIGHT HEART FAILURE

We subsequently carried out a prospective, multicenter study with 19 patients with decompensated right heart failure due to primary or secondary PH, with 79% of functional class NYHA IV, and 21% with the early signs of organ failure (kidney/liver)[18]. The baseline hemodynamics were seriously abnormal, with a mean PVR of 1804 dyne.s.cm^{-5}, a mean

TABLE 2 Treatment of a 45-year-old woman with primary pulmonary hypertension, with nitric oxide (NO) followed by inhaled iloprost. (a) Initial hemodynamic responses; (b) treatment for circulatory shock over the next 12 months[17]

(a)

	Admission		
	Base	NO	Inhaled iloprost
Pulmonary vascular resistance (dyn.s.cm^{-5})	2415	1920	1580
Systemic vascular resistance (dyn.s.cm^{-5})	2140	2050	1500
Pulmonary artery pressure (mmHg)	64	62	61
Systemic artery pressure (mmHg)	62	64	65
Pulmonary vascular resistance/ systemic vascular resistance	1.13	0.94	1.05
Cardiac output (l/min/m^2)	1.25	1.52	1.81

(b)

Parameter	Normal range	Admission	After 1 month	After 12 months
pO_2 (mmHg)	>78	51	65.4	66.3
Base excess (mmol/l)	0	-6.3	-2.5	-2.6
Creatinine (mg/dl)	0.7–1.3	1.8	1.1	0.9
Urea (mg/dl)	11–55	86	34	31
GOT (U/l)	6–18	680	14	14
GPT (U/l)	4–19	679	9	13
LDH (U/l)	140–240	2556	270	238
Bilirubin (mg/dl)	<1.1	5.2	2.5	1.5
6-min walk (m)		0	137	248

cardiac index of 1.6 l/min/m^2, and a low mean central venous oxygen saturation of 47%. We administered inhaled iloprost to these very ill patients in a non-controlled fashion for 3 months. In spite of treatment, four subjects died, three due to right heart failure. However, 43% of the patients improved considerably, moving up from NYHA class IV to class III. In parallel, their physical capacity, as measured by the 6-min walk test, improved significantly, even in some patients who were incapable of any exercise at baseline (Figure 6). Hemodynamics also improved, with the PAP falling, the cardiac index increasing and also the ratio PVR/SVR decreasing, indicating some preferential pulmonary vasodilator effect (Figure 7).

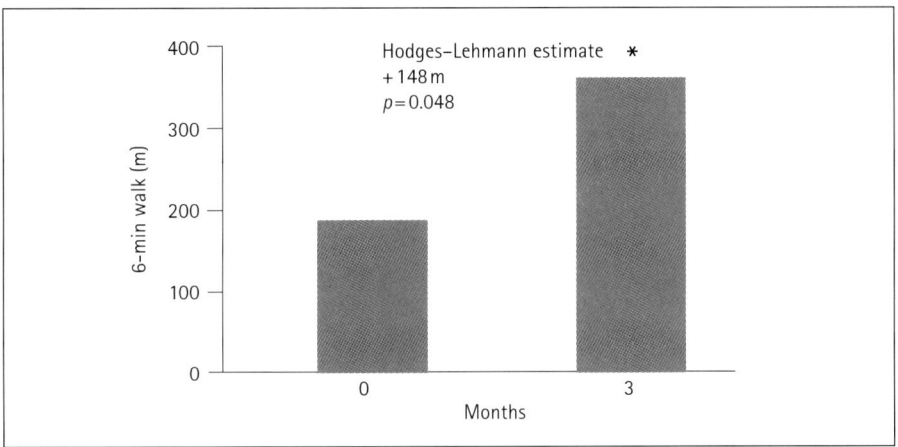

FIGURE 6   Effect of inhaled iloprost on exercise capacity in patients with decompensated right heart failure[18]

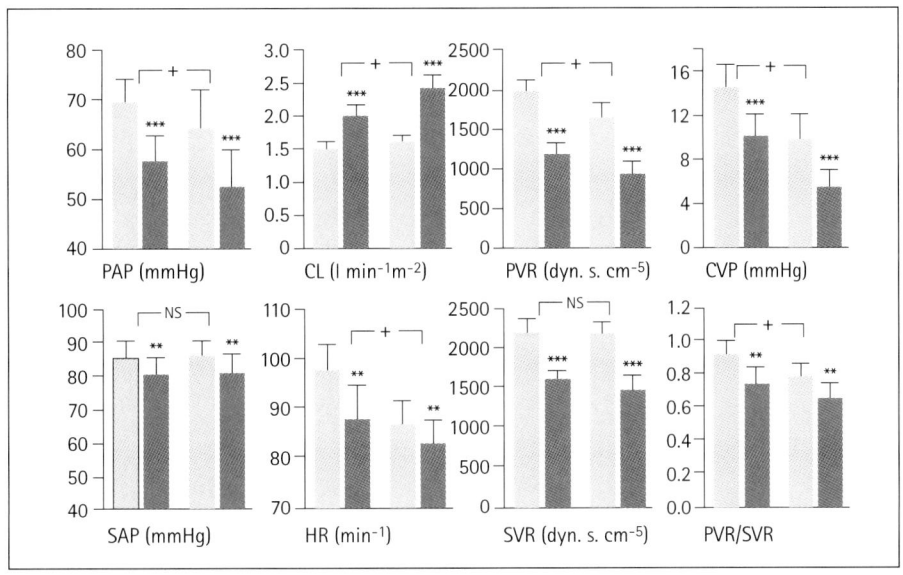

FIGURE 7   Effects of inhaled iloprost on cardiopulmonary variables in patients with decompensated right heart failure[18]

TREATMENT OF SEVERE LUNG FIBROSIS WITH PH WITH INHALED ILOPROST

Inhaled iloprost was next considered on a compassionate basis for another type of patient, as demonstrated in the first patient treated, a 27-year-old woman with mixed collagenosis and progressive lung fibrosis. She was breathless at rest, bedridden, and showed progressive digital acral necrosis. In addition to fibrosis, this patient had developed severe secondary pulmonary hypertension, with a baseline PAP of 65 mmHg and a PVR of 2243 dyne.s.cm^{-5}. She was treated with inhaled NO, intravenous prostacyclin and inhaled prostacyclin, responding very well to all three approaches (Table 3). However, the use of intravenous prostacyclin had the disadvantage that it markedly increased the shunt flow to 23.1%, which could not be tolerated by the patient, whereas there was only a minimal increase in shunt flow with NO and aerosolized prostacyclin. She has now been successfully treated with aerosolized prostacyclin for several years.

This single case was followed up with a study of all three treatments in eight patients with lung fibrosis and secondary pulmonary hypertension (Figure 8)[19]. All three agents caused a decrease in PAP, and there was a significant increase in cardiac output for intravenous and aerosolized prostacyclin, but not for inhaled NO. Both NO and aerosolized prostacyclin were associated with a decrease in PVR/SVR, indicating preferential pulmonary vasodilatation. In particular, in these fibrosis patients, the expected shunting of blood within the pulmonary vasculature occurred in response to intravenous prostacyclin, but only minor shunting was observed with aerosolized prostacyclin (Figure 9).

TABLE 3 Acute response to vasodilatory therapy in lung fibrosis with decompensated right heart failure

	CO (l/min)	PAP (mmHG)	PVR (dyn.s.cm^{-5})	RVEF (%)	CVP (mmHg)	HR (bpm)	MAP (mmHg)	paO$_2$ (mmHg)	Shunt (%)
Pre-NO	2.1	65	2243	7	18	113	110	69.4	3.6
During NO	5.0	44	774	15	10	90	120	88.6	6.3
Pre-PGI2 i.v.	2.4	59	1789	9	19	111	121	71.9	5.1
During PGI2 i.v.	6.0	42	470	20	10	102	105	62	23.1
Pre-PGI2 aero	2.5	65	2179	7	18	113	112	74.6	2.4
During PGI2 aero	4.7	45	644	20.5	9.5	93	113	81.5	5.6

CO, cardiac output; PAP, pulmonary artery pressure; PVR, pulmonary vascular resistance; RVEF, right ventricular ejection fraction; HR, heart rate in beats/min; MAP, mean arterial pressure; paO$_2$, arterial partial oxygen pressure; Shunt, shunt flow

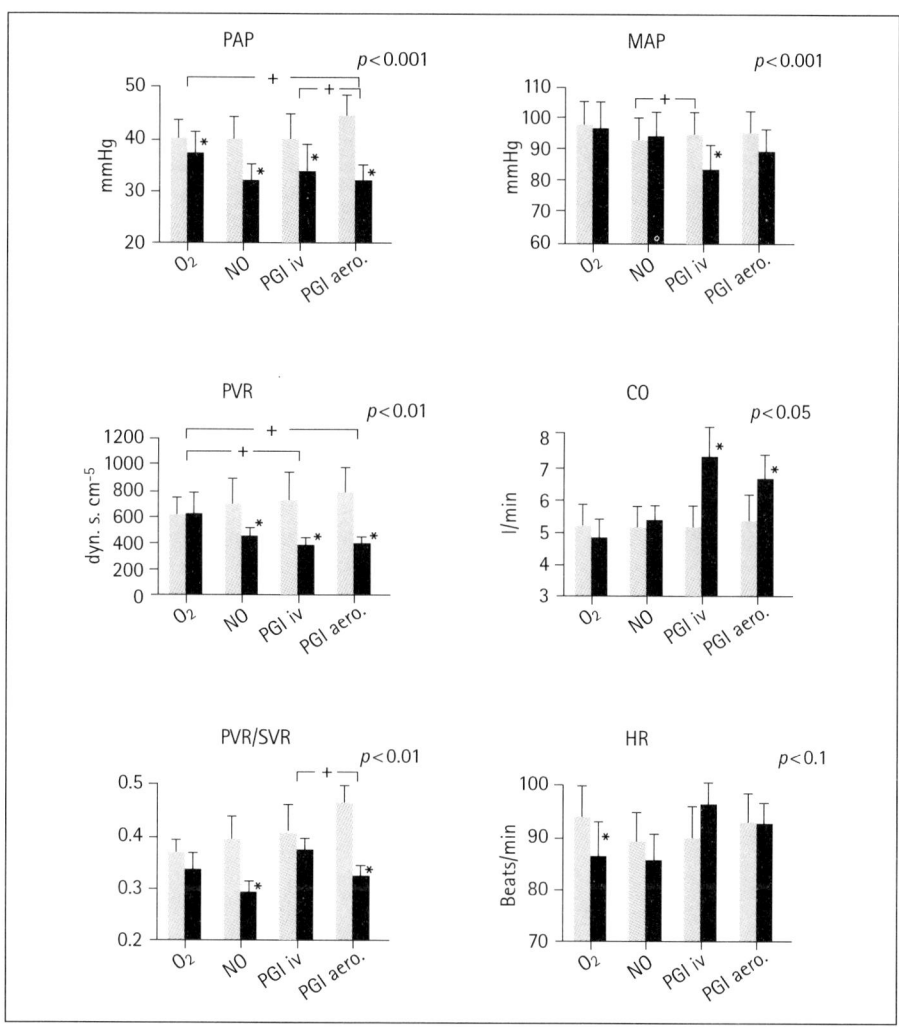

FIGURE 8 Comparison of the effects on cardiopulmonary variables of treatment with NO, inhaled and intravenous iloprost in a series of eight patients with severe lung fibrosis and pulmonary hypertension[19]

LONG–TERM OBSERVATIONS OF INHALED ILOPROST THERAPY

Inhaled iloprost therapy has now been observed clinically for 7 years[18,20,21]. The study by Höper and colleagues[20], which involved 23 patients with primary pulmonary hypertension, demonstrated a fall in PVR with aerosolized iloprost over a 12-month period (Figure 10) and a marked improvement in walking distance. A non-controlled study with aerosolized

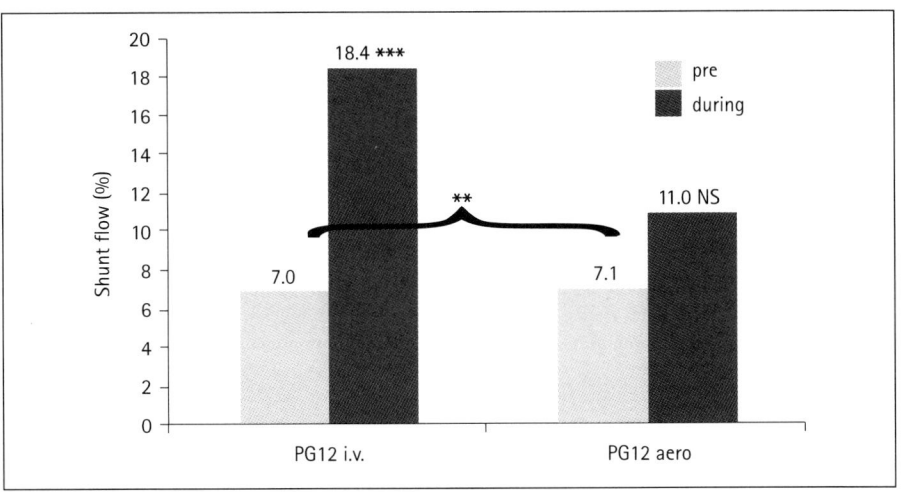

FIGURE 9 Data from a study of eight patients with severe lung fibrosis and pulmonary hypertension, showing the greater shunting of blood from the lungs with intravenous prostacyclin, compared with aerosolized delivery[19]. ***, $p < 0.001$ vs. baseline; **, $p < 0.01$ for change between baseline and drug

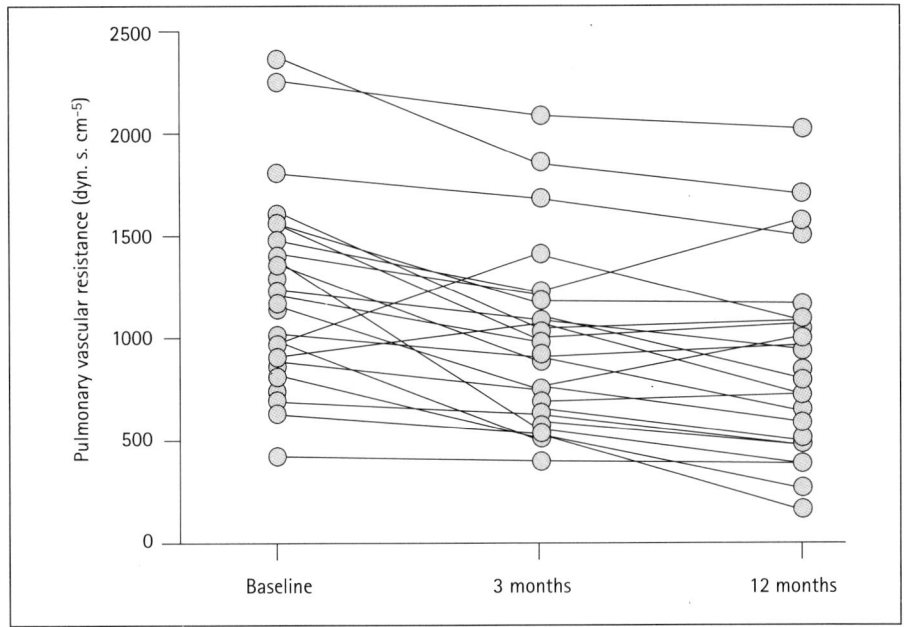

FIGURE 10 Changes in pulmonary vascular resistance with 12 months' treatment with aerosolized iloprost in primary pulmonary hypertension[18]

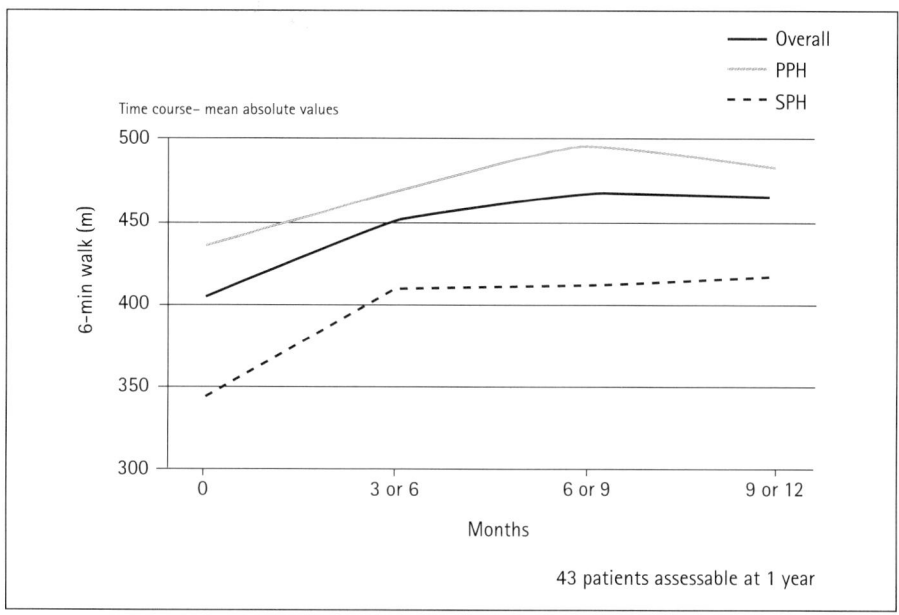

FIGURE 11   Effect of inhaled iloprost therapy on exercise capacity (6-min walk distance) over a 12-month period[21]

iloprost in 63 patients with primary and secondary pulmonary hypertension has also shown an improvement at 1 year, in all patients, of about 90 m in walking distance, based on data from 43 patients (Figure 11)[21].

COMPARISON OF INHALED AND INTRAVENOUS ILOPROST THERAPY

It is clear that there are some disadvantages to inhaled iloprost compared with intravenous therapy. Thus, it is necessary to use several inhalations per day, sometimes as many as 12. Each inhalation may last 10 min, though 4 min is more usual. Between inhalations, almost all the hemodynamic advantages of therapy are lost, resulting in a therapeutic gap, particularly during the night, although the significance of this is not clear. Occasionally, inhalation therapy is associated with transient respiratory tract irritation, but this is rarely significant. However, there are also many clear-cut advantages of inhaled iloprost. Thus, there are very few systemic side-effects, PAP is significantly reduced, there are no catheter complications, and only a very moderate degree of tachyphylaxis has been observed over a period of several years. Moreover, aerosolized iloprost is appropriate for treating both primary and secondary hypertension and it is also less costly than intravenous therapy.

REFERENCES

1. Barst RJ, Rubin LJ, McGoon MD, *et al.* Survival in primary pulmonary hypertension with long-term continuous intravenous prostacyclin. *Ann Intern Med* 1994;121:409–15

2. Barst RJ, Rubin LJ, Long WA, *et al.* A comparison of continuous intravenous epoprostenol (prostacyclin) with conventional therapy for primary pulmonary hypertension. *N Engl J Med* 1996;334:296–301

3. McLaughlin VV, Genther DE, Panella MM, Rich S. Reduction in pulmonary vascular resistance with long-term epoprostenol (prostacyclin) therapy in primary pulmonary hypertension. *N Engl J Med* 1998;338:273–7

4. Rich S, Kaufmann E, Levy PS. The effect of high doses of calcium channel blockers on survival in primary pulmonary hypertension. *N Engl J Med* 1992;327:76–81

5. Sitbon O, Humbert M, Jagot JL, *et al.* Inhaled nitric oxide as a screening agent for safely identifying responders to oral calcium channel blockers in primary pulmonary hypertension. *Eur Respir J* 1998;12:265–70

6. Channick RN, Newhart JW, Johnson FW, *et al.* Pulsed delivery of inhaled nitric oxide to patients with primary pulmonary hypertension: an ambulatory delivery system and initial clinical tests. *Chest* 1996;109:1545–9

7. Robbins I, Christman BW, Newman JH, *et al.* A survey of diagnostic practices and the use of epoprostenol in patients with primary pulmonary hypertension. *Chest* 1998;114:1269–75

8. Conte JV, Gaine SP, Orens JB, *et al.* The influence of continous prostacyclin therapy for primary pulmonary hypertension on the timing and outcome of transplantation. *J Heart Lung Transpl* 1998;17:679–85

9. Higenbottam T, Butt AY, McMahon A, *et al.* Long term intravenous prostaglandin (epoprostenol or iloprost) for treatment of severe pulmonary hypertension. *Heart* 1998;80:151–5

10. Jones RC. Role of interstitial fibroblasts and intermediate cells in microvascular remodelling in pulmonary artery hypertension. *Eur Respir Rev* 1993;3:569–75

11. Olschewski H, Seeger W. *Pulmonary Hypertension – Pathophysiology, Diagnosis, Treatment, and Development of a Pulmonary-selective Treatment*, 1 edn. Bremen, Germany: UNI-MED, 2002

12. Walmrath D, Schneider T, Pilch J, Grimminger F, Seeger W. Aerosolised prostacyclin in adult respiratory distress syndrome. *Lancet* 1996;342:961–2

13.   Walmrath D, Schneider T, Pilch J, Schermuly R, Grimminger F, Seeger W. Effects of aerosolized prostacyclin in severe pneumonia. Impact of fibrosis. *Am J Respir Crit Care Med* 1995;151:724–30

14.   Walmrath D, Schneider T, Schermuly R, Olschewski H, Grimminger F, Seeger W. Direct comparison of inhaled nitric oxide and aerosolized prostacyclin in acute respiratory distress syndrome. *Am J Respir Crit Care Med* 1996;153:991–6

15.   Olschewski H, Walmrath D, Schermuly R, Ghofrani A, Gimminger F, Seeger W. Aerosolized prostacyclin and iloprost in severe pulmonary hypertension. *Ann Intern Med* 1996;124:820–4

16.   Höper MM, Olschewski H, Ghofrani HA, *et al*. A comparison of the acute hemodynamic effects of inhaled nitric oxide and aerosolized iloprost in primary pulmonary hypertension. German PPH study group. *J Am Coll Cardiol* 2000;36:1440

17.   Olschewski H, Ghofrani HA, Walmrath D, Temmesfeld-Wollbruck B, Grimminger F, Seeger W. Recovery from circulatory shock in severe primary pulmonary hypertension (PPH) with aerosolization of iloprost. *Int Care Med* 1998;24:631–4

18.   Olschewski H, Ghofrani HA, Schmehl T, *et al*. Inhaled iloprost to treat severe pulmonary hypertension. An uncontrolled trial. German PPH Study Group. *Ann Intern Med* 2000;132:435–43

19.   Olschewski H, Ghofrani HA, Walmrath D, *et al*. Inhaled prostacyclin and iloprost in severe pulmonary hypertension secondary to lung fibrosis. *Am J Respir Crit Care Med* 1999;160:600–7

20.   Höper MM, Schwarze M, Ehlerding S, *et al*. Long-term treatment of primary pulmonary hypertension with aerosolized iloprost, a prostacyclin analogue. *N Engl J Med* 2000;342:1866–70

21.   Nikkho S, Seeger W, Baumgartner R, *et al*. One-year observation of iloprost therapy in patients with pulmonary hypertension. *Eur Respir J* 2001;18(Suppl 33):324s

DISCUSSION

Unknown questioner

Do you consider that, with the inhalation of prostanoid, there is absolutely no systemic effect, or do you consider that such a systemic effect is dose-dependent?

Professor Seeger

What is the local effect and what is the systemic effect? That is not so easily answered for the prostanoids as it is for NO. With NO the situation is clear, because it only has the chance to vasodilate as long as it is in the air space – when it enters the blood, it binds to hemoglobulin. Concerning the effects of aerosolized prostacyclin, we have experimental and clinical evidence.

As regards the experimental evidence, we have used wash-out, i.e. we had perfused lungs with no recirculation of the perfusate, which only allows a direct effect at the moment at which the drug enters the lung. We have compared the kinetics of entry into the perfusate volume as compared to the kinetics of vasodilation. From these experimental data, we feel that a large part of the effect is due to the local regional effect of the high concentration of drug being delivered down the alveolar space, but there is clear 'spill-over' and the effects of recirculating drug.

In the clinical studies, we always see with iloprost that, compared to intravenous prostacyclin, we have a decrease of the ratio PVR/SVR, which is not so marked as with NO, but is greater than that seen with intravenous prostacyclin. Hence, I would say that, with inhaled iloprost, we have two effects: a direct, local vasodilatory effect, but also spill-over into the general circulation that also contributes to the vasodilation.

In answer to your second question, the systemic effect is dose-dependent. Iloprost is not an ideal controlled-release drug so it passes into the circulation, and, when we increase the dose, there is more spill-over, leading to flushing in patients. This effect limits the escalation of dosage, since the systemic effects of flushing and headache become more obvious. The strategy we followed in all the initial studies was to determine a dose at which we have some of the initial systemic effects immediately after inhalation, but with a rapid levelling off of these effects for the convenience of patients. With a controlled drug delivery system, it might also be possible to have higher doses and a local effect, but without significant systemic effect.

6

Positive outcome of the Aerosolized Iloprost Randomized pivotal study in primary and non–primary pulmonary hypertension

H. Olschewski

Iloprost is a stable prostacyclin analog with a half-life substantially longer than the natural compound. Delivered directly to the lungs as an aerosol, iloprost has been shown to exert selective pulmonary vasodilatation, with few side-effects (as discussed in Chapter 5). In brief, several pilot studies (Table 1)[1–8] have shown that aerosolized iloprost improves physical capacity and cardiopulmonary hemodynamics in patients with severe pulmonary hypertension (PH) and related conditions. Two studies (Table 1)[9,10] have shown a negative result with similar therapy, although it is not possible to exclude the possibility that these used suboptimal doses of inhaled iloprost, since the nebulizers used had not been physically characterized. In order to test the findings of these non-controlled studies, a placebo-controlled trial of the use of inhaled iloprost has now been carried out, the Aerosolized Iloprost Randomized (AIR) pivotal study, the results of which are reported in this chapter.

The AIR study builds on clinical observations of compassionate treatment given since 1994, which showed encouraging outcomes, together with clinical developments carried out by Schering AG (Berlin, Germany), including a long-term surveillance study (SAG 98008)[1], and an open-label study carried out over 2 years in Germany[11]. Most recently, Behr and colleagues[12] have shown the consistency of the acute hemodynamic response to inhaled iloprost in patients with PH over a 12-month period and Nikkho and colleagues[11] have

TABLE 1   Analysis of results in previous studies on inhaled iloprost

Reference	Patients	Nebulized iloprost (µg)	Inhaled iloprost (µg)	Observation period	Result
Favorable results					
1–3	Crest, PPH, LF	100–150	18–36	1 year	improved
4	5 severe PH	100	18	5 months	improved
5	19 severe PH	50–200	9–36	3 months	improved
6	24 PPH	100–150	18–36	1 year	improved
7	51 severe PH	100	18	≤ 2 years	stabilized, safety
8	63 severe PH	100–200	18–45	1 year	improved, safety
Unfavorable results					
9	3 patients on i.v. PGI2	150–300	?	≤ 2 weeks	deterioration
10	12 severe PH	100 (–150)	?	3–19 months	deterioration

demonstrated the excellent safety profile of long-term use of inhaled iloprost therapy in such a setting.

THE INHALED DOSE: NEBULIZER STUDIES

All the non-controlled studies of iloprost were carried out with a special nebulizer (the Ilo-Neb®), which is very easy and safe to use, but which has the disadvantage that the delivered dose is unpredictable, since it depends on the ventilatory pattern of the patient. Studies showed that administering a nebulized dose of 9–15 µg of iloprost with the Ilo-Neb device resulted in a mean inhaled dose (the amount delivered to the patient) of 2.8 µg, but there was a large variation, up to a maximum inhaled dose of 6.7 µg. Clearly, it is important to know the inhaled dose of iloprost delivered to patients, since it is likely to be critical to the success or otherwise of such therapy. Before starting the AIR study, it was, therefore, decided to investigate the pharmacokinetics of iloprost and its hemodynamic effects when delivered by three different devices in a group of 12 typical PH patients (SAG 98051)[13]. The trial was an open-label, randomized, three-period, cross-over design. The aim was to deliver inhaled doses in the upper range of those given during empiric therapy, namely, 5 µg with each of the devices and to compare the effects.

It was recognized that there may be important differences between inhalation devices, so the nebulizers used in the comparison study (HaloLite™, Ventstream™, and IloNeb®) were chosen to exemplify very different techniques for targeting the alveoli, even though they were all set to deliver 5 µg of iloprost to the mouthpiece of the device. All three nebulizers yielded the same hemodynamic and pharmacokinetic outcomes in the patients[13]. In the pharmacokinetic study, the first of its kind for iloprost, the measured peak serum levels of the drug were found to be close to those achieved with intravenous administration. However, the serum half-life was very short, ranging from 6.5 to 9.4 min, depending on the inhalation device used. Significantly, the half-life of hemodynamic effects is longer (21–25 min) than that of the drug, presumably due to local deposition and local action of iloprost, with recirculation of the drug playing only a minor part in its action.

For the AIR study, we selected the Halolite™ nebulizer (MedicAid, Sussex, UK) which targets the alveoli and is technically very efficient, but which has the additional advantage that it provides exact dosing, by computing the delivered dose and ceasing delivery at a predefined level. As well as giving confidence in the delivered dose, this particular nebulizer minimized drug wastage. It was a compressor-driven jet device, delivering aerosol pulses when triggered to do so by the patient's inspiration.

The inhaled doses used in the AIR study were in the range of several published non-controlled studies in which favorable outcomes were reported (Table 1). These demonstrated that, for successful treatment, patients required two to three ampules of iloprost per day, involving a daily nebulized dose of 100–150 µg (in some cases up to 300 µg) and an inhaled dose of 18–45 µg (about 60 µg maximum).

THE AEROSOLIZED ILOPROST RANDOMIZED PIVOTAL STUDY

Method

The AIR study (SAG 97218) involved 203 patients with primary and non-primary pulmonary hypertension (NYHA classes III and IV), recruited from 37 specialized centers throughout Europe[14]. Patients were randomized to 12 weeks' therapy with inhaled iloprost or placebo, followed by a 4-week observation period. Patients were stratified for underlying disease and NYHA class. Entrance to the study required that the patients had primary pulmonary hypertension or selected forms of non-primary pulmonary hypertension, including that associated with collagen vascular disease and appetite suppressants as well as non-operative chronic thromboembolic pulmonary hypertension. Their NYHA functional class was III or IV despite standard conventional therapy, and their capacity on the 6-min walk test was 50–500 m. The major exclusion criteria were severe obstructive or restrictive lung disease, acute or chronic inflammatory lung disease, pulmonary venous congestion, congenital heart disease, pregnancy or insufficient contraceptive measures, or previous therapy with prostaglandins. The patients recruited to the AIR study (Table 2) were about 50 years of age, predominantly female, as expected, with about equal numbers having severe primary and non-primary PH, mainly with a chronic thromboembolic etiology. Interestingly, more than half the patients were receiving oral vasodilator therapy, but none of them were receiving high-dose calcium channel blockers. Although a large number of patients were in functional class NYHA III, this study involved more patients in NYHA class IV than any previous study (Table 3). Baseline hemodynamic data (Table 4) confirmed that patients had severe pulmonary hypertension, with a mean pulmonary artery pressure (PAP) of about 53 mmHg, a pulmonary vascular resistance (PVR) in excess of 1000 dyne.s.cm^{-5}, and a central venous oxygen saturation level (measured during long-term oxygen administration) of about 60%.

Iloprost dosing

The study protocol allowed the nebulized iloprost dose to be titrated during the first 8 days, according to determined regimens (Table 5). Most patients used the maximum (nebulized)

TABLE 2   Anthropometric data. Unless otherwise stated, data are presented as number of cases (%)

	Iloprost	Placebo
Age (years)	51.2 (1.31)	52.8 (1.19)
Weight (kg)	71.3 (1.45)	72.6 (1.37)
Male/female (%)	31.7 / 68.3	33.3 / 66.7
Underlying disease		
PPH	51 (50.5)	51 (50.0)
NPPH	50 (49.5)	51 (50.0)
appetite suppressants	4(4.0)	5 (4.9)
collagen vascular disease	13 (12.9)	22 (21.6)
CTEPH	33 (32.7)	24 (23.5)
Oral vasodilator therapy	52 (51.5)	58 (56.9)

PPH, primary pulmonary hypertension; NPPH, non-primary pulmonary hypertension; CTEPH, chronic thromboembolic pulmonary hypertension

dose of 5 µg per inhalation, with about half undertaking six inhalations per day and the others nine inhalations per day. The mean nebulized dose was 37.5 µg/day, which translates into the relatively low dose rate of only 0.37 ng/kg/min. Normal dose rates for intravenous iloprost are 2–10 ng/kg/min and for intravenous prostacyclin 10–100 ng/kg/min.

Primary and secondary endpoints

The primary endpoint of the study was a combined clinical endpoint, consisting of an improvement of at least one functional class, at least a 10% improvement in the 6-min

TABLE 3   Functional capacity. Data are presented as number of cases (%) or mean ± SEM

	Iloprost	Placebo
NYHA functional class		
II	60 (59.4)	59 (57.8)
III	41 (40.6)	43 (42.2)
Mahler Dyspnea Index score	4.14 ± 0.18	4.27 ± 0.18
6-min-walk (m)	332 ± 9	315 ± 10

TABLE 4   Hemodynamics. Data are presented as mean ± SEM

	Iloprost	Placebo
Pulmonary artery pressure (mmHg)	52.8 (1.15)	53.8 (1.41)
Cardiac output (l/min)	3.8 (0.11)	3.8 (0.09)
Pulmonary vascular resistance (dyn.s.cm^{-5})	1029 (41)	1041 (50)
Systemic vascular resistance (dyn.s.cm^{-5})	1872 (67)	1827 (54)
CPR (mmHg)	9.2 (0.54)	8.2 (0.51)
PAWP (mmHg)	7.5 (0.37)	7.6 (0.45)
SaO_2 (%)	92.6 (0.54)	92.2 (0.59)
SvO_2 (%)	60.4 (0.82)	60.5 (0.89)
Heart rate (beats/min)	83.9 (1.23)	81.8 (1.56)

TABLE 5   Possible titrations of iloprost dose during the first 8 days for the highest tolerated dose

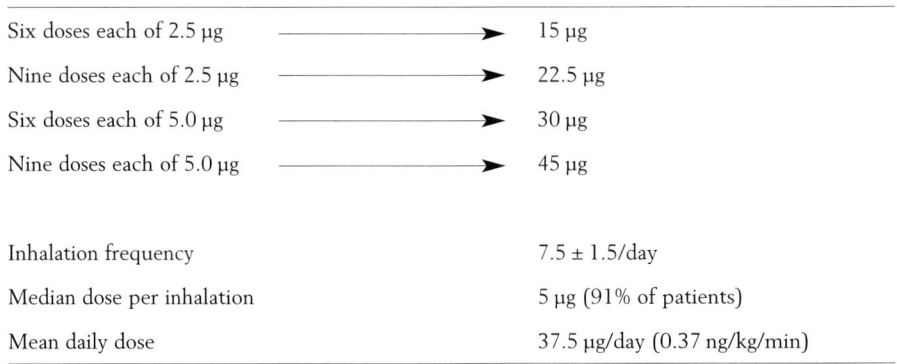

Six doses each of 2.5 µg	→	15 µg
Nine doses each of 2.5 µg	→	22.5 µg
Six doses each of 5.0 µg	→	30 µg
Nine doses each of 5.0 µg	→	45 µg
Inhalation frequency		7.5 ± 1.5/day
Median dose per inhalation		5 µg (91% of patients)
Mean daily dose		37.5 µg/day (0.37 ng/kg/min)

walking test, no deterioration, and no death. Secondary endpoints were the 6-min walking test, NYHA class, Mahler Dyspnea Index, hemodynamic parameters, defined criteria of deterioration, and quality of life.

Results

Clinical outcome

The proportions of patients who improved their exercise capacity and NYHA class, and also those who reached the combined clinical endpoint, are shown in Figure 1, which demonstrates a highly significant advantage of inhaled iloprost over placebo ($p = 0.007$). It is interesting to note a relatively high placebo response in the 6-min walk test, which is probably due to the relatively high variance of this measure. The placebo response was much lower for NYHA functional class, and very few patients in the placebo group attained the combined clinical endpoint. Looking in detail at the data for changes in NYHA class (Table 6), it can be seen that one patient in the iloprost group improved by two classes, although the majority improved by only one class. There was no significant difference in the numbers of patients who deteriorated in the iloprost and placebo groups, but, looking at the worst end of the scale, there were more patients who prematurely withdrew consent for the study in the placebo group (4 vs. 14), mainly because they did not experience any benefit from the treatment, and there were also more deaths in the placebo group (1 vs. 4), although the numbers in these comparisons were too small to prove statistical significance.

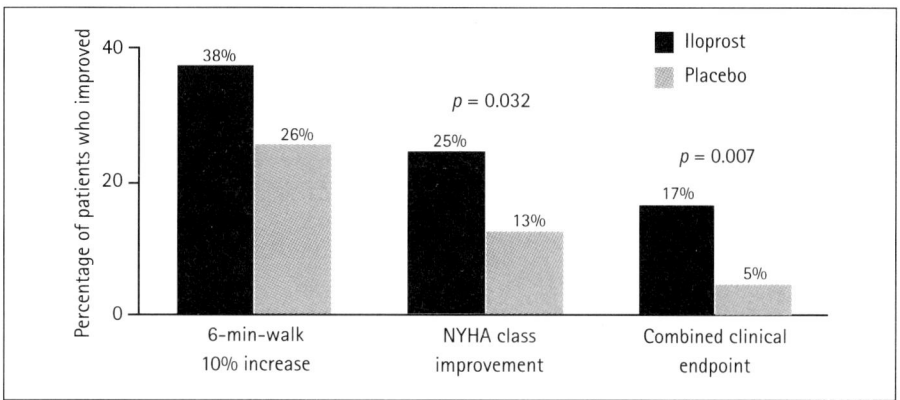

FIGURE 1 Major clinical outcomes in the AIR study (% of patients who improved), demonstrating a statistically significant difference for inhaled iloprost over placebo for NYHA functional class and the combined clinical endpoint

TABLE 6 Change in NYHA class. Data are given as number of cases (%)

NYHA class change	Iloprost	Placebo
Improved by 2 classes	1 (1.0%)	0
Improved by 1 class	24 (23.8%)	13 (12.7%)
Unchanged	65 (64.4%)	67 (65.7%)
Deteriorated	6 (5.9%)	8 (7.8%)
Missing data	1	0
Premature end of study	4 (4.0)	14 (13.7%)
death	1 (1.0)	4 (3.9%)
other	3	10

Exercise capacity and quality of life

Over the 12 weeks of therapy, exercise capacity according to the 6-min walk test improved significantly for the iloprost group, compared to placebo, with a clear gap after 4 weeks that widened with time (Figure 2). Patients were asked at the end of the study whether they felt better after the treatment, and their responses formed the basis of the Mahler Dyspnea Transition Index (Figure 3)[15], which showed a highly significant benefit for inhaled iloprost.

Another quality of life index, the EuroQol Visual Analog Scale (Figure 4)[16], was also measured. It had a scale from zero, meaning 'I couldn't feel worse' to 100, meaning 'I couldn't feel better.' Values at baseline were similar in the two groups, but, after 12 weeks' treatment, there was a significant improvement in the inhaled iloprost group, compared with a slight deterioration in the placebo group.

Cardiopulmonary hemodynamics

Over the 12 weeks of the study, the trough values of PAP in the placebo group and in the iloprost group did not change, but there was a significant reduction of about 4 mmHg after iloprost inhalation (Figure 5a). There was a slight improvement in the trough values of cardiac output in the inhaled iloprost group, compared with a deterioration with placebo and a significant improvement after inhalation (Figure 5b). Most importantly, the PVR increased in the placebo group, showing a significant difference to the inhaled iloprost group (Figure 5c).

Outcomes by subgroup

The study outcomes were analyzed for different groups of patients, who were stratified in terms of primary and non-primary pulmonary hypertension, and also according to NYHA functional class. This analysis showed no significant difference between the subgroups in

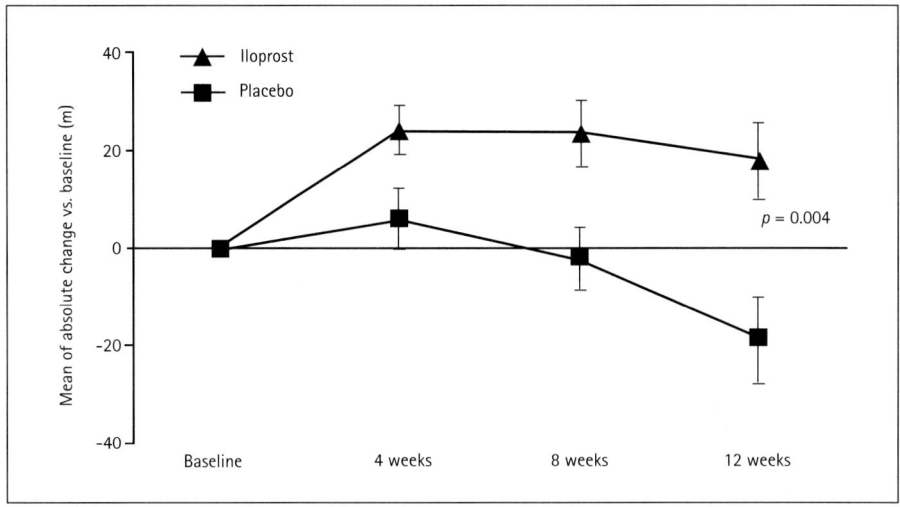

FIGURE 2   Exercise capacity according to the 6-min walk test at various time points in the AIR study, showing an advantage, widening with time, for inhaled iloprost over placebo

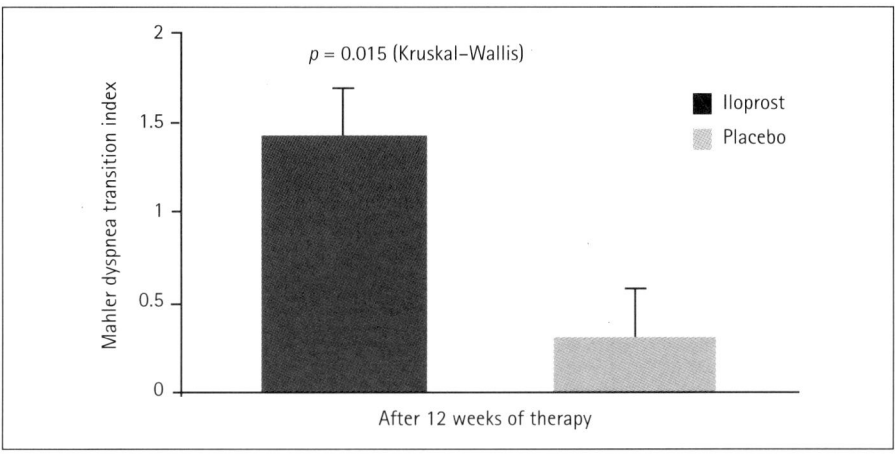

FIGURE 3 Data for the Mahler Dyspnea Transition Index in the AIR study, showing a significant advantage for inhaled iloprost over placebo

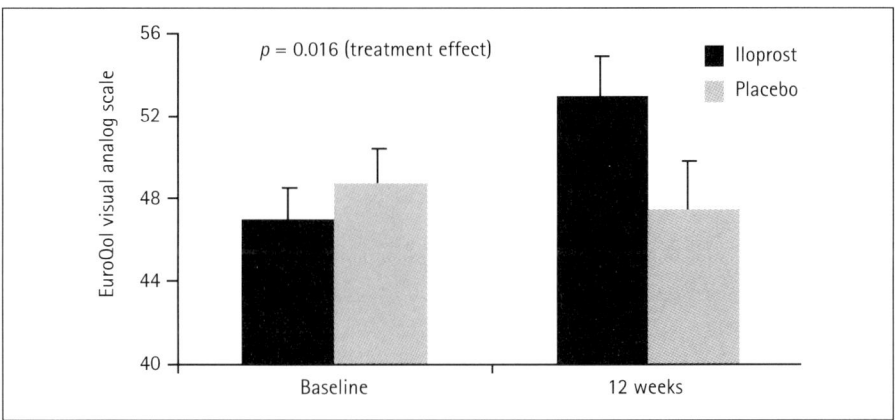

FIGURE 4 Pre- and post-study values of the EuroQuol Visual Analog Scale in the AIR study, showing an improvement in the quality of life experienced by those on iloprost, but not placebo

terms of the Mahler Dyspnea Transition Index, all patients responding to inhaled iloprost (Figure 6). Carrying out a similar analysis for exercise capacity according to the 6-min walk test, there was a clear difference between the iloprost and placebo groups for primary PH, but not for non-primary PH, which is difficult to explain (Figure 6). However, analysis with the combined clinical endpoint, which includes the 6-min walk data, showed a benefit of

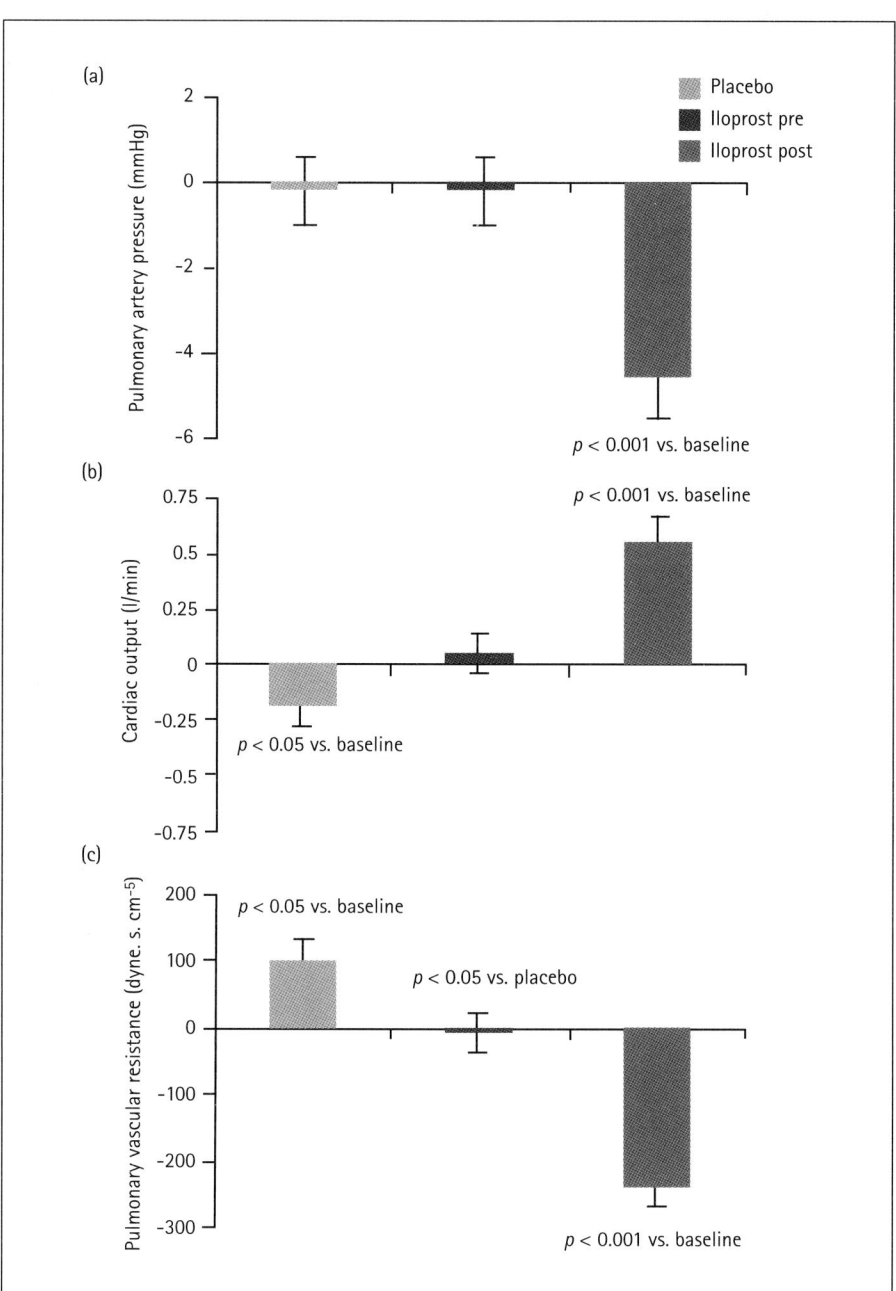

FIGURE 5 Hemodynamic changes measured over the 12 weeks of the AIR study. (a) Mean pulmonary artery pressure (PAP) demonstrated a significant decrease with inhaled iloprost therapy, but not with placebo; (b) cardiac output significantly improved with iloprost but not with placebo; (c) pulmonary vascular resistance significantly decreased with iloprost but not with placebo

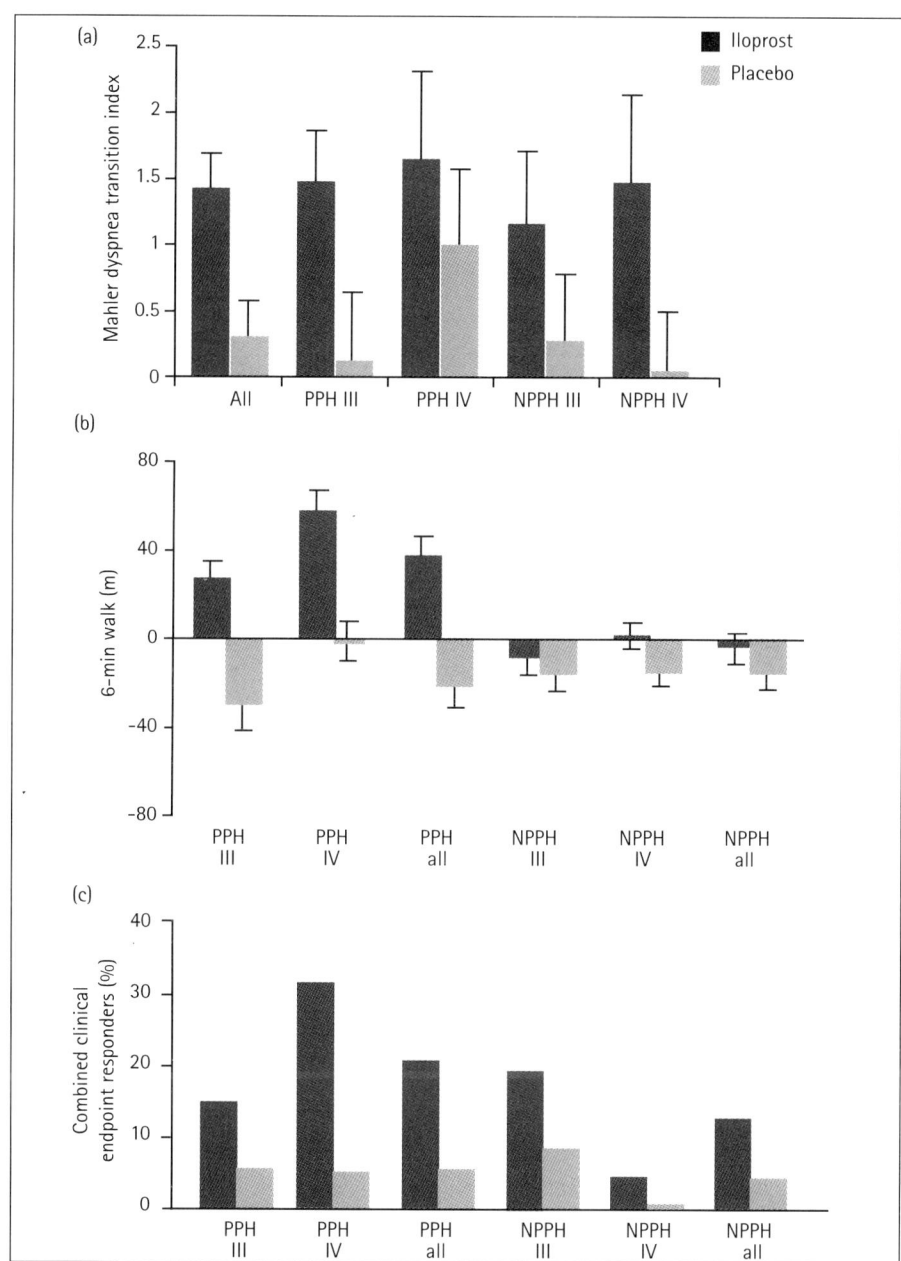

FIGURE 6 Subgroup analysis in the AIR study. (a) All subgroups responded to inhaled iloprost, with no significant differences between the subgroups in terms of the Mahler Dyspnea Transition Index; (b) in the 6-min walk test, patients with primary pulmonary hypertension (PPH) showed significant improvement but those with non-primary pulmonary hypertension (NPPH) did not; (c) for the combined clinical endpoint, all subgroups showed significant improvement with inhaled iloprost

inhaled iloprost for patients with both primary PH and non-primary PH, and there is, therefore, no reason to suppose that the treatment is ineffective for non-primary PH (Figure 6).

SAFETY

Serious adverse events during the AIR study, that were life-threatening and/or required hospitalization, are shown in Table 7. There were more cases of heart failure in the placebo group than the inhaled iloprost group (8 vs. 3). Headache, flushing and influenza-like symptoms, which are typical of intravenous prostanoids, were not noted as serious adverse events in this study. There were more cases of syncope rated as serious adverse events with inhaled iloprost therapy than with placebo (5 vs. 0), although two of the patients with syncope were responders in terms of the combined clinical endpoint and none experienced a deterioration in their clinical state. Moreover, data for all adverse events (Table 8) showed no significant difference in incidence of syncope in the two groups. Obviously, for whatever reason, the episodes of syncope in the iloprost group were more often considered to be more severe than those in the placebo group. Data for all adverse events also showed that, as would be expected, flushing and jaw pain were more common in the inhaled iloprost group. Most of the adverse events were mild and transient.

TABLE 7   Serious adverse events. Data are given as number of cases (%)

	Iloprost	Placebo
Heart failure	3 (3.0)	8 (7.8)
Increased cough	0	0
Headache	0	0
Flush	0	0
Flu syndrome	0	0
Periphal edema	0	2 (2.0)
Nausea	1 (1.0)	1 (1.0)
Trismus	0	0
Hypotension	2 (2.0)	1 (1.0)
Diarrhea	1 (1.0)	0
Syncope	5 (4.9)	0
Vertigo	0	0

TABLE 8   Adverse events. Data are presented as number of cases (%)

	Iloprost	Placebo
Increased cough	39 (38.6)	26 (25.5)
Headache	30 (29.7)	20 (19.6)
Flush	27 (26.7)	9 (8.8)
Flu syndrome	14 (13.9)	10 (9.8)
Peripheral edema	13 (12.9)	16 (15.7)
Nausea	13 (12.9)	8 (7.8)
Jaw pain	12 (11.9)	3 (2.9)
Hypotension	11 (10.9)	6 (5.9)
Diarrhea	9 (8.9)	11 (10.8)
Syncope	8 (7.9)	5 (4.9)
Vertigo	7 (6.9)	11 (10.8)

CONCLUSIONS

The AIR study has proven that inhaled iloprost is effective in the treatment of severe PH, including disease due to chronic thromboembolism, which is difficult to treat. A noteworthy feature of the study is that it is the first of its kind to have included a significant proportion of patients with a poor functional class (NYHA IV), who have hitherto been regarded as unlikely candidates for inhaled iloprost therapy. The results of the AIR study demonstrate that even such patients, with poor functional class, can derive benefit from this therapy. The administration of aerosolized iloprost proved to be safe, without toxic effects on the liver, lung, or kidney, and its use obviated the catheter complications that are typical of intravenous administration of the drug. The AIR study has shown inhaled aerosolized iloprost therapy for severe pulmonary hypertension to be effective and extremely well tolerated, in comparison with other methods of delivering prostanoids, due, no doubt, to the selective pulmonary effects that can be achieved by directing iloprost to the focus of the condition. It combines the well-established benefits of prostacyclin with pulmonary selectivity, without any evidence of tachyphylaxis over the 12-week period of the study.

REFERENCES

1.   Olschewski H, Walmrath D, Schermuly R, *et al.* Aerosolized prostacyclin and iloprost in severe pulmonary hypertension. *Ann Intern Med* 1996;124:820–4

2.   Olschewski H, Ghofrani HA, Walmrath D, *et al.* Recovery from circulatory shock in severe primary pulmonary hypertension (PPH) with aerosolization of iloprost. *Intensive Care Med* 1998;24:631–4

3.   Olschewski H, Ghofrani HA, Walmrath D, *et al.* Inhaled prostacyclin and iloprost in severe pulmonary hypertension secondary to lung fibrosis. *Am J Respir Crit Care Med* 1999;160:600–7

4.   Stricker H, Domenighetti G, Fiori G, *et al.* Sustained improvement of performance and haemo-dynamics with long-term aerosolised prostacyclin therapy in severe pulmonary hypertension. *Schweiz Med Wochenschr* 1999;129:923–7

5.   Olschewski H, Ghofrani HA, Schmehl T, *et al.* Inhaled iloprost to treat severe pulmonary hypertension. An uncontrolled trial. German PPH Study Group. *Ann Intern Med* 2000;132:435–43

6.   Hoeper MM, Schwarze M, Ehlerding S, Adler-Schuermeyer A, Spiekerkoetter E, Niedermeyer J, et al. Long-term treatment of primary pulmonary hypertension with aerosolized iloprost, a prostacyclin analogue. *N Engl J Med* 2000;342:1866–70

7.   Ewert R, Opitz C, Wensel R, *et al.* [Iloprost as inhalational and intravenous long-term treatment of patients with primary pulmonary hypertension. Register of the Berlin Study Group for Pulmonary Hypertension]]. *Z Kardiol* 2000;89:987–99

8.   Nikkho S, Seeger W, Baumgartner R, *et al.* One-year observation of iloprost therapy in patients with pulmonary hypertension. *Eur Respir J* 2001;18(Suppl 33):324s

9.   Schenk P, Petkov V, Madl C, *et al.* Aerosolized iloprost therapy could not replace long-term IV epoprostenol (prostacyclin) administration in severe pulmonary hypertension. *Chest* 2001;119:296–300

10.   Machherndl S, Kneussl M, Baumgartner H, Schneider B, Petkov V, Schenk P, *et al.* Long-term treatment of pulmonary hypertension with aerosolized iloprost. *Eur Respir J* 2001;17:8–13

11.   Nikkho S, Seeger W, Baumgartner R, *et al.* One-year observation of iloprost inhalation therapy in patients with pulmonary hypertension. *Eur Respir J* 2001;18:324s [abstract]

12.   Behr J, Baumgartner R, Borst M, *et al.* Consistency of the acute hemodynamic response to inhaled iloprost in pulmonary hypertension patients treated with long-term iloprost aerosol. *Eur Respir J* 2001;18:323s [abstract]

13. Olschewski H, Rohde B, Behr J, Ewert R, Gessler T., Ghofrani HA, *et al.* Comparison of inhalation of the prostacyclin analogue iloprost using different nebulizer systems in patients suffering from pulmonary hypertension. *Chest* 2000;118(Suppl):136s

14. Olschewski H, Simonneau G, Nazzareno G, *et al.* Inhaled iloprost for severe pulmonary hypertension. *N Engl J Med* 2002;347:322–9

15. Mahler DA, Weinberg DH, Wells CK, *et al.* The measurement of dyspnea. Contents, interobserver agreement, and physiologic correlates of two new clinical indexes. *Chest* 1984;85:751-758

16. EuroQol – a new facility for the measurement of health-related quality of life. *The EuroQol Group. Health Policy* 1990;16:199–208

DISCUSSION

Unknown questioner

If I remember correctly, in your original studies in the mid-1990s, you used 20 µg of iloprost for each dose but now you use only 5 µg. Why is this?

Dr Olschewski

The inhaled dose and the nebulized dose are quite different. In previous papers, we gave the nebulized dose, i.e. the dose you put into the nebulizer, but the patients only inhale a part of this, in the proportion of about 1 : 3.

Unknown questioner

So the amount put into the nebulizer was the same, about 20 µg?

Dr Olschewski

Yes, this is true. In this study we used a different nebulizer, which was filled so that it delivered an inhaled dose of 2.5 or 5.0 µg of iloprost to the patient.

Professor Higenbottam

There is a very important message here. It is important to use precise dosing with all these therapies.

Dr Kneussl

Thank you very much for presenting our data in one slide. However, concerning our patients, we received the same advice from Schering, using the same tool for administration, and we followed your protocol for the dosage. We used the same pressure and the same influx. However, from the clinical point of view, our patients all required intravenous epoprostenol [prostacyclin] and they rejected it and so we administered iloprost by inhalation. But I think we need to discuss the data and consider any differences between our studies.

Dr Olschewski

This is an unsolved question, to determine what really made the difference between the observations made by your group and others. As you mentioned, patient selection – which seemed to be a negative selection in your group for inhaled iloprost – played a big role. And you did not use the physically characterized inhalation devices in all your patients.

Professor Higenbottam

We can go through the two studies, but I refer the questioner to an excellent Editorial in the same journal written by one of our speakers, Dr Nazzareno Galiè, that makes the point that, with all these therapies, unlike 15 years ago, when treatments were being tried in small series of patients, we now have randomized controlled trials.

Dr Popov (Switzerland)

I would like to speculate on the fact that the patients in the iloprost group had more syncope. Probably, these patients were in a better condition for taking exercise and therefore they had the opportunity to generate syncope, but this is easy to review if patients are questioned.

Dr Olschewski

Indeed, there is some indication that these patients were more active than they should have been. Nearly all these instances of syncope occurred long after the last inhalation, so may be these patients did too much exercise and should have rested and taken another inhalation.

Professor Mayer (Mainz, Germany)

I was a little surprised that more than 30% of your patients had chronic thromboembolic pulmonary hypertension (CTEPH), and I would like, from the surgical point of view, to state that there is a potentially curative alternative for these patients in terms of surgery, and at this time almost all the patients with CTEPH can be operated on with a reasonable risk.

Professor Higenbottam

These patients had peripheral thrombotic disease. To emphasize a point that Dr Nazzareno Galiè has made, and we have also heard at one of our previous symposia, we do not yet know the relative risk of doing surgery compared with not doing it, because there has been no trial.

Dr Olschewski

These CTEPH patients were all considered to be non-operable at specialized centers. A large proportion of these patients were enrolled in Paris, where they have a lot of experience with arterectomy. So I do not think that many of these patients could have been operated on.

Dr Sofi (Naples, Italy)

Have you any imaging data for the distribution of iloprost in the respiratory tract, for example, using scintigraphy?

Dr Olschewski

There are some data, and we are doing more studies in order to develop better inhalation devices for a more homogenous deposition of the drug. It is not easy.

Professor Nazzareno Galiè (Bologna, Italy)

You have shown hemodynamic data at baseline and at the end of the inhalation therapy. So the data are for all the patients, both those treated with placebo and iloprost?

Dr Olschewski

Yes, all available data from the placebo and the iloprost groups were included. The data presented were changes from baseline. This means that all the patients who had two catheter investigations were included.

Professor Galiè

Yes, my question is: In the vasoreactivity test, we performed a treatment. Do you notice any difference between the patients treated with placebo and iloprost?

Dr Olschewski

No, there was no difference in the acute vasoreactivity during inhalation of iloprost comparing patients that had been on 12 weeks of placebo and those on iloprost.

Professor Galiè

For hemodynamics, there was no change at baseline and no change after vasoreactivity testing in both groups, placebo and iloprost?

Dr Olschewski

Baseline hemodynamics deteriorated in the placebo group and were unchanged in the iloprost group. This difference between groups was significant for PVR, for instance.

Unknown questioner

The lack of therapy at night-time did not appear to be a clinical problem.

Dr Olschewski

Right. There was not a single patient who had a major problem with the cessation of therapy through the night.

Professor Higenbottam

One of the surprising details in this is the dose of the prostanoid that the patients were receiving, which was surprisingly low. You also showed us the pharmacokinetic curve, which showed that people only achieved the equivalent serum level of the intravenous dose for a very short time. And yet, as you have shown, there was a longer-lived effect in the circulation. This goes some way to answer Dr Simonneau's earlier question about, in part, iloprost acting locally within the lung, though there is still a sharp spike within the serum which may account for some of the high levels of flushing observed. Is that a valid interpretation?

Dr Olschewski

That's absolutely true. We also saw in the device comparison studies some correlation between systemic side-effects and the plasma levels, but not between plasma levels and hemodynamic effects. So this is another indication that the local effects are more important.

Professor Higenbottam

I would like to ask Dr Simonneau what the circulating level of beraprost sodium was in that study in relation to the level we see with intravenous prostanoids.

Professor Simonneau

We have pharmacokinetic data from about 12 patients, six with primary pulmonary hypertension and six with secondary disease. In the primary group, the peak concentration [of beraprost] was about 400 pg/ml, and in the secondary group it was about 100 pg/ml. The reason for the difference is that the patients with primary pulmonary hypertension have a very low clearance rate, although the reason for this is not clear.

Professor Sean Gaine (Dublin, Ireland)

We heard earlier that intravenous prostacyclin was developed as a bridge to transplantation. What do you think of the proposition that, from the data you have shown, aerosolized iloprost is a bridge to intravenous prostacyclin therapy? Would you let a patient deteriorate on inhaled iloprost without giving them the option of intravenous therapy?

Dr Olschewski

In our practice, we have seen many patients with inhalation therapy as primary therapy. And, within this group, there are some who are stable over a long period and who do not need any further therapy. There are others who deteriorate, despite inhalation therapy, and at some point need additional therapy. Normally, we use additional intravenous iloprost for these patients, with good results.

Professor Galiè

Iloprost is a very good tool for testing for acute vasoreactivity, and we have shown that, in many cases, you can reduce PVR by about 50%. In these patients, the WHO guidelines say that we need to use calcium antagonists. What should we do when we observe acute vasoreactivity with iloprost? Should we first use oral calcium antagonists and then see whether we can obtain a further effect with iloprost, or should we give iloprost first, as for your first patient 7 years ago, who was a responder and in many other centers would have been treated with calcium antagonists.

Dr Olschewski

You would have killed her! I agree the inhaled iloprost test is safe and gives very large responses from the pulmonary vasculature. However, we do not use it to test for calcium channel responses. Instead, we use the inhaled NO test, as described by Olivier Sitbon from Professor Simonneau's group, because only those patients who respond to the latter test have a good chance of being good responders to calcium antagonists. Many more patients will respond to inhaled iloprost, but their chances of being good responders to calcium antagonists are very low.

Professor Galiè

So your suggestion is to use NO for acute vasoreactivity?

Dr Olschewski

Yes, at least for identification of the best patients. The weaker compound finds out the good candidates for high-dose calcium channel blockers.

Dr Groves (Denver, Colorado, USA)

I appreciate very much your data and am impressed with the results, but when we had intravenous iloprost available in the late 1980s/early 1990s, after we had had a lot of experience with intravenous prostacyclin as an acute hemodynmaic challenge, we then used intravenous iloprost in 26 patients and we found very comparable results with iloprost to that which we had had with intravenous prostacyclin. We had published data to support the concept that, in our center, a combination of a greater than a 30% drop in PVR and a greater than 10% drop in mean PAP could be used to define responders. In those responders, we were able to show that they did respond to calcium channel blockers, both acutely and chronically. So I would differ with your interpretation.

Dr Olschewski

I think there's much inhomogeneity between centers. I know that most German centers use inhaled NO, probably also the French. The Americans use either prostacyclin as an acute infusion, or adenosine. Hardly anyone uses calcium antagonists, because they are too dangerous for acute testing. Nobody has ever tried to put these data together, in order to really define how the good responders to calcium channel blockers can be identified in an optimal way.

Professor Higenbottam

Dr Groves did it actually, but we could not persuade Dr Rich, the editor of the WHO guidelines, of the validity of the work. I suspect that, with the very high lung levels of drug that you can achieve by inhalation, you are looking at a very different sort of mechanism. I'm sure you're right, Bert, and we did try to argue very fiercely for the standards you had set.

Dr Groves

Just for clarification, if you use NO as an acute test and you find significant vasoreactivity, according to defined parameters, do you give those patients a trial of calcium channel blockers, or do you put them on inhaled iloprost, which I think would be a considerably more complicated therapy, and possibly more expensive, although I don't know anything about the costs?

Dr Olschewski

If we find a patient who responds well to inhaled NO, and has a PVR lower than 800 dyne.s.cm^{-5}, during NO inhalation, this is normally a reduction of PVR of more than 30%, then we start a therapy with high-dose calcium channel blockers as first-line therapy.

Dr David Lyon (Dublin, Ireland)

I work for the Irish national and the European regulatory authorities and I have been interested in the recruitment problem when we discuss clinical trial plans with companies. We are usually told that there are not enough patients. Now, from the number of studies which have been reviewed this evening, I'm beginning to think that there may be a problem recruiting patients with PH who have not been previously treated and there is also the consideration that, when these products are licensed, it looks as if it is going to be unethical not to treat patients, so there will be an even more complicated problem in the future. I do not often have the opportunity to have a pool of investigators together like this and so I cannot resist raising a rather philosophical question. Do any of the speakers have any comments on the issue?

Professor Seeger

This is, indeed, a serious question. I think many of us will feel that the period when we did treatment versus placebo in patients with pulmonary hypertension is now over. We now clearly have tools in our hands for those patients not on intravenous prostacyclin, and, in, say, a year's time, it will not be possible to make comparisons with placebo. We then have to make another step, but what should we do? To compare therapy A with therapy B, B against C, or to combine treatments? I really would strongly support trials of combinations, because we have to be aware that, even with the best results we have, with the exception of a small proportion of patients, pulmonary artery pressures will not be brought within the normal range. For most patients I think we will need combination therapy to achieve optimal effects.

Professor Higenbottam

I think that is probably a good final word on the subject, because many of the patients will die despite treatment, and one is trying to buy the best optimal care in the earliest instance for most of the patients. So, I suspect that what Dr Seeger is saying is true, that people would prefer to add in an existing therapy and do the comparison in that sort of way.

Index